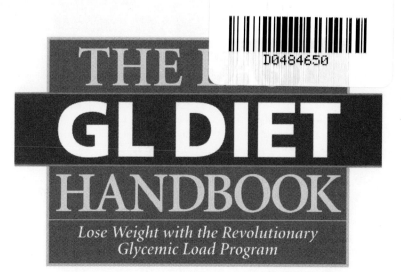

THE NEW
GL DIET
HANDBOOK

Lose Weight with the Revolutionary
Glycemic Load Program

Dr. Fedon Alexander Lindberg

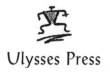

Ulysses Press

Published in the U.S. by Ulysses Press
P.O. Box 3440
Berkeley, CA 94703
www.ulyssespress.com

First published as *Beyond GI: Understanding Glycaemic Load* in Great Britain in 2006 by Rodale International Ltd.

ISBN10: 1-56975-574-4
ISBN13: 978-1-56975-574-7
Library of Congress Control Number 2006907918

Printed in Canada by Transcontinental Printing

10 9 8 7 6 5 4 3 2 1

Proofreader: Elyce Petker
Production: Matt Orendorff
Cover design: Double R Design

Distributed by Publishers Group West

This book has been written and published strictly for informational purposes, and in no way should be used as a substitute for consultation with health-care professionals. You should not consider educational material herein to be the practice of medicine or to replace consultation with a physician or other medical practitioner. The author and publisher are providing you with information in this work so that you can have the knowledge and can choose, at your own risk, to act on that knowledge. The author and publisher also urge all readers to be aware of their health status and to consult health-care professionals before beginning any health program.

Contents

Introduction

Ever since my first book was published in Norway in 2001, a silent revolution has taken place there. A staggering 24 percent of the Norwegian population have changed their dietary habits and turned to the balanced, slow-carb, good-fat Mediterranean-inspired diet that I advocate. *The Easy GL Diet Handbook* provides a quick and easy introduction to the principles of my diet, and provides all the information you need to choose foods—and in particular, carbohydrates—wisely.

If you have picked up this book, you are probably familiar with the Glycemic Index (GI), a method of ranking foods according to how quickly they raise the blood sugar. Numerous books advocating a low-GI diet have appeared in recent years, many of which seem to contradict the previous generation of diet books. For more than 30 years, nutritionists were convinced that if you wanted to lose weight, all you had to do was reduce your fat intake; carbohydrates were not a problem. Scientific research has found that not all carbohydrates are equal, even though they provide the body with the same amount of energy: measured in calories, carbohydrates have 4 calories per gram. In fact, the effect one carb source has on blood sugar can be strikingly different from another. Some are digested and absorbed slowly, leading to a gentle rise in blood sugar, while others are absorbed quickly, causing a sharp rise in blood sugar—the quicker the rise in blood sugar, the higher the GI.

Why is this information so important? Because, in short, our blood sugar levels are closely connected with hunger, cravings and the extent to which we store or burn fat. Put simply, if a carbohydrate has a high GI it will raise the blood sugar rapidly and provide lots of energy that, if it isn't used, will be stored as fat. There is one major problem, however: GI can be misleading, because it is always measured by testing 50 grams of carbohydrate, not 50 grams of food. Although GI tells you how fast 50 grams of carbohydrate in a particular food raises your blood sugar, it gives no clue as to the effect of the portion you actually eat. To get 50 grams of carbohydrates you need to eat 50 grams of glucose or sugar, but over 19 pounds of oranges.

This is why the Glycemic Load (GL) is now widely regarded as a more accurate measure. GL is, in the same way as the GI, an index ranking foods according to their effect on blood sugar. But while GI gives us information on how fast blood sugar rises after we eat 50 grams of digestible carbohydrate in various foods, the GL takes into account both the GI and the amount of carbohydrate in 100 grams of food or a given portion and therefore reflects the amount of carbohydrate we actually eat.

It is important to bear in mind that GL is not the only health measure. If it were, margarine, with a GL of 0, would be extremely healthy—but we all know it is not. This book will help you to understand healthy fats and proteins, as well as carbs, because a healthy diet is a balanced diet: neither low-fat nor low-carb is a sensible way to lose weight and stay healthy. The Easy GL Diet is all about balance, combining the latest in scientific research with the traditional wisdom of the Mediterranean diet, and in this book you will find plenty of information to help you choose wisely when shopping and eating out, as well as extensive GI and GL lists for easy reference.

Read, understand, eat and enjoy the healthy life!

Essentials:
Why Your Body Needs This Book

During recent years, the incidence of so-called lifestyle diseases such as obesity and diabetes has been increasing at an alarming rate. As a doctor with a family history of diabetes I developed an early interest in this area. A predisposition for disorders such as obesity, diabetes, high blood pressure and high cholesterol are known to be genetically inherited, but lifestyle is what determines who will become ill and when. Therefore my interest was personal as well as professional—I wanted to know what I could do to avoid becoming one of the statistics.

Until a few years ago, the only medicines available to treat diabetes increased the body's production of insulin (the hormone responsible for regulating blood sugar levels, which is already high in the early stages of type II diabetes and in most cases of obesity). These medicines improved the control of blood sugar levels, but almost without exception they led to weight gain, increased blood pressure and increased levels of triglycerides and cholesterol in the blood.

In many cases, insulin-injection treatment would become necessary a few years down the line, resulting in even further weight gain. The obvious conclusion: Too much insulin makes us fat!

What affects our insulin levels? The answer is very simple: the food we eat—not so much the quantity we eat, but what we choose to eat.

While working in the United States in the 1990s, I came across two terms that have had a great impact on many people around the world: Glycemic Index (GI) and Glycemic Load (GL). The Glycemic Index is a scientific method that measures the effect of carbohydrates on blood sugar levels; Glycemic Load relates the GI to the amount of carbohydrate eaten in a normal serving, or in 100 grams (which makes comparison between foods possible). The right carbohydrates, coupled with the right quality and quantity of proteins and beneficial fats, will allow your body to reach a healthy balance. I soon realized that this was one of the most important milestones in modern nutrition. Used correctly, this nutritional principle can prevent and counteract a wide range of health problems.

Are you overweight?

A low-glycemic diet is especially suitable for anyone who has a tendency to put on weight easily, especially around the waist, or who is already overweight or obese. If you have been overweight for a number of years or have tried countless diets, only to regain all the weight you lost, do not despair. You have not necessarily gained weight because you eat too much, but mainly because you eat the wrong food. By choosing the right food—and with a little bit of planning—you can lose weight permanently while eating well and becoming healthier with every bite.

Are you predisposed to heart disease?

If you have high blood pressure, elevated cholesterol or triglyceride (blood lipid) levels, or have already developed angina or had a heart attack or stroke, it is more than likely that food has contributed to your problems. Along with quitting smoking, mastering stress, sleeping well and leading a physically more active life, a low-glycemic diet will have an enormous impact on your health. It can improve your blood pressure, reverse atherosclerosis and even open up nearly blocked arteries. Our body has a fantastic ability to heal itself, if only it is given the chance.

Are you predisposed to diabetes?

If you have diabetes in your immediate family, eating a low-glycemic diet can greatly reduce your chances of getting the disease yourself. If you are one of the 190 million people in the world with type II diabetes (adult-onset diabetes), you can achieve better control of your blood-sugar levels and prevent a series of complications related to this disease (the damage it causes to blood vessels and nerves can result in blindness, amputation, impotence, kidney disease, heart disease and stroke).

According to Centers for Disease Control and Prevention, more than 80 percent of people diagnosed with type II diabetes are overweight. If you are among that group, a low-glycemic diet will help you gradually lose excess body fat.

If you have type I diabetes, you will find you have steadier, more predictable blood sugar and the need for insulin will be reduced, although you will still be dependent on insulin shots; you will also avoid developing complications linked to the disease, which are caused by poor blood sugar control.

Do you have insulin resistance?

How can you tell if you have insulin resistance? The easiest way is simply to look at yourself in the mirror. If your belly is bulging even though the rest of your body looks normal, then you are probably predisposed to hyper-insulinemia (increased production of insulin) and you may have already developed insulin resistance (impaired insulin action). If you are very overweight or obese, you almost certainly are insulin-resistant. The same is true if you have type II diabetes or if your doctor has tested your cholesterol levels and found you have increased triglycerides and reduced HDL ("good") cholesterol. High blood pressure is another likely indicator.

Even if you are of a normal weight and shape, you may have insulin resistance; in the developed world around 10 percent of the population have insulin resistance without any other health or weight problems. Insulin resistance can develop into syndrome X, also called metabolic syndrome, a hormonal disorder that puts you at increased risk of type II diabetes, obesity, heart attack, stroke and several forms of cancer, as well as inflammatory diseases.

Some of us have a genetic predisposition to becoming insulin-resistant, but our eating and exercise habits determine whether or not we actually develop the syndrome. So the answer is clear—change your habits and change your life.

Stressed out?

Warning: Stress can seriously damage your health. In nature, acute stress is a necessary survival reaction, but the chronic stresses of modern life have nothing to do with real danger—you can't run away from them! So the hormones that nature intended to help us deal with stress remain in the bloodstream, causing chronic stress, with symptoms such as weight gain, low libido, difficulty in concentrating and poor memory, as well as more serious problems.

Stress often affects the way we eat: we skip meals, or turn to "comfort food." But the high-carb, high-fat foods we generally choose as "comfort" send our blood sugar soaring then plummeting. Unfortunately, the body interprets rapidly falling blood sugar levels (which also occur when we skip meals) as a stressful situation and secretes even more stress hormones. By avoiding foods that send our blood sugar on a rollercoaster ride we can begin to tackle this vicious cycle of chronic stress.

Always tired and sluggish?

Have you been feeling abnormally tired and sluggish for a long time? Do you lack concentration and feel irritable? This may be due to a hormonal imbalance caused by your diet and lifestyle. Today's foods are a far cry from what we are genetically designed to eat, and some individuals tolerate a modern diet better than others. Foods that cause a rapid increase in blood sugar—high-GI/GL foods—cause a corresponding sharp increase in insulin (the hormone that controls blood sugar levels), followed by a rapid drop in blood sugar. When this happens, you will probably feel tired, irritable, hungry and lacking in concentration.

The answer is to eat differently. You will enjoy increased mental alertness if you choose more natural whole foods that have a low GI/GL, such as vegetables and fruit, and increase your intake of foods containing omega-3 fats (the latter have been shown to elevate mood).

Do you crave certain foods?

Are you one of those people who craves sweets, bread or other types of starchy food? When you start eating something sweet, or a savory snack like potato chips, do you find you can't stop until you've finished the whole pack? After lunch you feel tired, even lethargic, your concentration is poor and you may become irritable. You grab some chocolate, or maybe a sweet drink, feel better quite quickly and have more energy, but an hour or two later you feel tired and hungry again. If this sounds familiar, it is possible that you are a carbohydrate addict.

Sugar addicts and anyone who is stressed or depressed are likely to turn to chocolate or other sweet and fatty or starchy foods because, by increasing the levels of serotonin and endorphins in the brain, they provide a soothing and calming effect. But they also cause high insulin levels, which can lead to obesity, type II diabetes, high blood pressure and cardiovascular disease.

By learning a little more about the way food and hormones such as insulin work together in your body, you can control your cravings—rather than have them control you.

Do you suffer from an inflammatory condition?

Inflammation is a natural part of the body's repair function, but when the inflammation process becomes chronic it causes disease. Inflammatory diseases—such as dermatitis, psoriasis, migraine, osteoarthritis, asthma, intestinal disorders and certain types of heart disease—have increased dramatically over the past 50 years, in parallel with the increased consumption of junk food, trans fats, refined carbohydrates and sugars, and the decline in consumption of natural whole foods. The good news is that by reducing our intake of high-glycemic carbohydrates, omega-6 fats and trans fats and increasing our intake of foods high in omega-3 fats (see page 36), together with antioxidant-rich foods, we can correct the balance and reduce inflammatory problems.

A diet for everyone

You need not be overweight or have a medical problem in order to be interested in achieving optimal health and vitality. Low-glycemic foods and the correct balance of nutrients are of equal importance for everyone. Over millions of years, our bodies have evolved to handle natural whole foods, not the highly processed food of our modern diet, which contains high levels of high-glycemic carbs and unhealthy, unnatural fats. We are what we eat—our bodies are literally made from the food we eat—so we need the right type of food in adequate quantities in order to be healthy. This book will help you make the right choices so that you and your family can feel full of energy and glow with health.

Understanding GI and GL

GI and insulin—the vital equation

To understand how eating low-glycemic foods can help you lose weight and become healthier, you need to understand the connection between GI and the hormone insulin.

Every time you eat foods containing carbohydrates (like bread, potatoes, rice, pasta, sugar and, to a lesser extent, vegetables, fruit and legumes), your blood sugar (also known as blood glucose) rises. The Glycemic Index is a method of ranking foods according to their impact on blood sugar—the more quickly a carbohydrate raises your blood sugar, the higher its GI.

As the blood sugar level rises, the pancreas secretes insulin, which is responsible for storing glucose from the bloodstream in the cells. Because the blood sugar level in the body needs to be kept within strict boundaries, the higher the rise in blood sugar the more insulin is released to deal with it. A limited amount of glucose can be stored in the liver and muscles (as glycogen)—any remainder is stored as fat. So quite simply, the more insulin you have in your blood, the more fat will be stored.

Besides making it almost impossible to lose weight, too much insulin can also result in long-term damage to your body. The more often your body experiences a high level of insulin, the more difficult it becomes for insulin to lower blood sugar. The pancreas tries to compensate for this by secreting more insulin. The more high-glycemic food you consume, the more insulin your body will produce, and as a result you soon become caught in a vicious circle of hyperinsulinemia (higher insulin production) and reduced insulin sensitivity (insulin resistance). When this happens, your insulin level remains high constantly, whether you have eaten or not. However, it is only the blood-sugar-lowering effect of insulin that has deteriorated. Insulin still continues to promote fat storage. The result is you will gain weight and have a greater risk of developing type II diabetes, high cholesterol levels, high blood pressure and cardiovascular disorders, as well as certain types of cancer.

No GI or a low GI isn't necessarily good

Foods that do not contain carbohydrates do not have a direct influence on blood sugar, consequently their GI is zero. This is why there are no GI numbers for foods that consist primarily of protein, such as eggs, chicken, meat and fish. The same is true of foods that consist mainly of fat, such as butter, margarine and oils. However, having a GI of zero does not mean a food is healthy. It is important to note that the GI does not tell you anything about the qualities of the food other than its impact on blood sugar. Some really unhealthy food have a low GI.

Of course there are plenty of good foods that do not have a GI rating. Apart from healthy proteins, there are a number of non-starchy vegetables that are not included in the GI lists. This is because such vegetables—tomatoes and celery are good examples—have a very low carbohydrate content, usually less than 5 percent, and you would therefore need to eat a lot of them in order to ingest the 50 grams of carbohydrate needed to measure their GI (GI ratings are based on the effect of 50 grams of any given carbohydrate). For this reason, you will not find the GI of many vegetables in the lists at the back of this book.

Glycemic Load—taking the GI a step further

It is tempting to take a Glycemic Index list and say that all food with a high GI is unhealthy, but the truth is always more complicated. If we concentrate solely on what is good or bad for your blood sugar—ignoring vitamins, minerals and fat for the moment—the amount of carbohydrates eaten is clearly important. However, the GI is a measure of how fast the carbohydrate in any given food raises blood sugar; it does not take into account the amount of carbohydrate contained in the food (i.e., how much of it you would need to eat to elicit the response suggested by its GI). Remember, the amount of insulin produced is based on the amount of carbs as well as how fast they are converted to blood sugar (blood glucose).

Researchers from Harvard University have therefore come up with the Glycemic Load (GL). Introduced in 1997, it is now recognized as a more accurate way of expressing the glycemic effect of foods. The GL is, in the same way as the GI, an index ranking foods according to their effect on blood sugar. However, while GI gives us information on how fast blood sugar rises after we eat 50 grams of digestible carbohydrate in various foods, the GL takes into account both the GI and the amount of carbohydrate in 100 grams of food or a standard portion. It therefore gives a far more accurate assessment of foods because it reflects the *amount* of carbohydrate we are consuming.

You will find a detailed list of foods and their GI and GL at the end of this book.

The use of the GL principle means that a number of foods that were effectively blacklisted (as far as their effect on blood sugar was concerned) under the GI system now appear in a far more favorable light. Watermelon is a good example. It has a GI of 72 because the carbohydrate it contains is high GI, but because it contains very little of that carbohydrate it has a GL per 100 grams of only 4. You would have a similar rise in blood sugar from eating 1000 grams (more than 2 pounds) of watermelon as you would from eating 100 grams (3½ ounces)—about 3 slices—of white bread, which has a GI of around 70. Another healthy food whose GI could lead us to believe it should be avoided is boiled carrot. It has a high GI but its GL per 100 grams is just 4.

What is high GL and what is low GL?

I would say that a GL of 20 or more is high, 11 to 19 is medium, and 10 and below is low. It is important to note that you should not get hung up on the exact GL number. It is much better to instead think of carbohydrates as high, medium or low glycemic. As a rule, foods with a low GL are a good choice, but there are always exceptions, especially foods that are high in saturated fat. You should think carefully before you eat food with a high GL (ideally none at all if you wish to lose weight) and stick to food with a

THE DIFFERENCE BETWEEN GI AND GL

Looking at the Glycemic Load per 100 grams of food allows you to compare foods in a way that is familiar from nutrition information labels. But remember that a normal serving may be more—or less—than 100 grams.

FOOD	GI	GL/100g
Glucose	100	100
Cornflakes	81	70
Sugar	68	68
White bread	70	36
Sourdough bread	54	25
Fructose	19	19
Baked potato	85	17
Spaghetti	39	10
Chickpeas	28	6
Boiled carrots	58	4
Watermelon	72	4
Lentils	26	3

medium or, better still, low GL. However, this does not mean you need to become a fanatic. Eating small amounts of a favorite high-GL food as part of a reward meal once in a while will not pose a major problem and may actually make it easier to stick to a balanced diet in the long run.

If you wish to compare the GL and GI of foods—an interesting exercise in uncovering which healthy foods fall foul of the GI rating—a GI of above 55 is considered high, 35 to 55 is medium and below 35 is low.

The GL of the food you eat

The lists at the back of this book give the GI and GL of hundreds of foods; GL has been calculated per 100 grams, to make it easier to compare foods in the same way that you do when looking at a nutritional information label. But it is equally important to consider the amount one normally eats. Pasta has a lower GL than white bread per 100 grams, but whereas 100 grams of bread is a reasonable serving, with a high GL of 36, very few people would eat just 100 grams of cooked pasta (GL 10)—a regular serving of cooked pasta is often closer to 200 grams, which would have a a GL of 20. All-Bran breakfast cereal has a relatively high GL of 21 per 100 grams, but an average 40-gram serving would give an acceptably low GL of 8.

The calculation of GL in a meal

OK, so you can find the GL of carrots. But it is not often that you eat carrots on their own. What really counts is the GL of the whole meal. It is possible to calculate the GL of a meal, but this is a task better suited to an experienced nutritionist than to the average layperson.

You can assume that if all the ingredients have a low GL, then the whole meal will, too. This is the safe way to go if you want to lose weight. However, it is possible to combine ingredients with a low GL with small amounts of high-GL ingredients and end up with a medium-GL meal.

The Easy GL Diet

Low-GL foods play a vital part in the diet I recommend but it is important to see them as part of the "bigger picture" of a healthy diet. Technically I call my diet the isoglycemic diet (*isos* is the Greek word for "equal"): It is all about balance. The aim is to restore a more natural balance of the types of carbohydrates, proteins and fats you eat, which will lead to more stable blood sugar, a reduction in body fat and better hormonal balance in your body. Improved hormonal balance leads to a better immune system, less joint pain, better skin, and fewer allergies or asthmatic conditions, plus improved mental and physical performance.

However, this is not a quick-fix diet intended for a short period of time. It is a nutritional concept you can and should follow for the rest of your life. If you are overweight you should not expect to lose more than 2–3 pounds per week; if you lose more than this it will affect your fat-free (muscle) mass, which is not good because it is muscle that keeps your metabolism active. This level of weight loss may seem slow to some, but by following these guidelines you will experience increased feelings of well-being and vitality that will stimulate you to continue.

The basics of the diet

I recommend that approximately one-third of your total energy intake (by which I mean calories, not amount of food) should come from low- and medium-glycemic carbohydrates: these are carbohydrates that don't make your blood sugar rise rapidly. Less than one-third should come from high-quality animal and plant proteins, and the rest from minimally processed natural fat, primarily monounsaturated and polyunsaturated fats, but also, to a lesser degree, saturated fats. Sounds too much like science? Don't worry, you do not need to count grams, percentages or calories. Naturally slim people do not count the calories they

THE FOOD TRIANGLE OF THE EASY GL DIET

A simple way to visualize this way of eating is to use a food triangle. Foods are positioned according to their GI, GL and overall health benefits—the higher up the triangle a food is, the less of it you should eat.

Saturated fat: butter, cheese

Sugar, white bread, white flour, potatoes

Unsaturated fat: olive oil, canola oil, nuts and seeds, oily fish

Durum wheat pasta, non-sticky rice (e.g., basmati, long-grain), whole-grain products, dense bread made from less processed grains

Protein: fish, chicken, meat, game, eggs, yogurt, cottage cheese

Vegetables, beans, low-glycemic fruit

eat, and neither need you. The palm of your hand is all you need to judge the amount of food you should eat, as I'll explain below.

To make this diet easy to follow, I've created what I call the ABC of the Easy GL Diet (see "plate model" opposite). Most of your meals will consist of approximately one-third protein foods and two-thirds low-glycemic carbohydrates. One meal a day—your "reward" meal—may consist of one-third protein, half low-glycemic carbohydrates and one-sixth medium- or high-glycemic carbohydrates. You can choose whether to have this for your breakfast, lunch or dinner. To be in tune with human metabolic biorhythm, it is probably best to have your reward meal as your breakfast or lunch, but many people will choose dinner, for practical and social reasons.

How much should I eat?

Without weighing and measuring, the diagrams on pages 25 and 26 will help you to gauge what your meals will look like. For an adult, the amount of protein food (meat, fish, chicken, eggs, cottage cheese, tofu) should be about as big and thick as the palm of your hand. Palm size varies from one person to another and is proportionate with the rest of the body. This is the amount of protein-based food (cooked and ready to eat) that you need, and it constitutes the A part of each of your three main meals.

The B part (mainly vegetables and legumes, as well as low-glycemic fruits and berries) should be twice as big as the protein part: two palms.

As for the C part of the reward meal, it should not be bigger than half a palm, and the B part should not be reduced to less than one and a half palms. Part C also includes dessert and cheese or wine/alcohol. While a glass of wine with your lunch or dinner is fine in terms of health, if you are trying to lose weight I recommend that you avoid alcohol or that you use it as the C part of your reward meal.

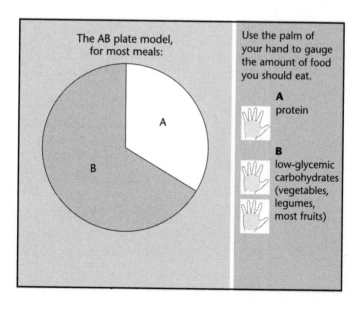

The AB plate model, for most meals:

A

B

Use the palm of your hand to gauge the amount of food you should eat.

A
protein

B
low-glycemic carbohydrates (vegetables, legumes, most fruits)

Snacks should be about half to one-third the size of main meals, keeping otherwise to the proportions.

Remember not to eat too quickly as it takes 10–15 minutes for satiety signals to reach the brain. If you feel you need a second helping, that's perfectly OK, but don't just eat more carbohydrates (such as rice, pasta, potatoes or bread). You must always balance what you eat so have

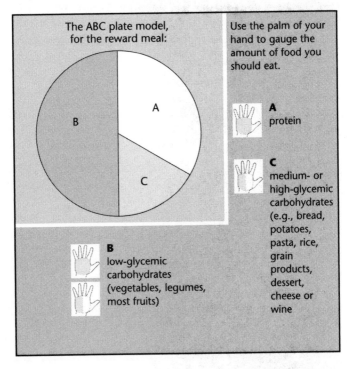

The ABC plate model, for the reward meal:

A

B

C

Use the palm of your hand to gauge the amount of food you should eat.

A
protein

C
medium- or high-glycemic carbohydrates (e.g., bread, potatoes, pasta, rice, grain products, dessert, cheese or wine

B
low-glycemic carbohydrates (vegetables, legumes, most fruits)

a corresponding (smaller) amount of protein (such as chicken, fish, meat, cottage cheese or yogurt). No meal or snack should be without protein.

Choosing the right foods

The Easy GL Diet is all about making the right food choices. The following section explains why particular elements of the diet are so important and which foods are best for your blood sugar—and your overall health.

Protein

Protein is crucial to our bodies. Our cells, hormones and immune system are all based on and communicate through proteins, so obviously we must ensure that we get enough of this nutrient. There are two sources of protein: animal protein and plant protein. Animal protein is found in milk and other dairy products, eggs, all meats, poultry, fish and shellfish. Note, it is the saturated fat in dairy products and meat that may be less healthy in large quantities, not the protein! If you choose lean meats and low-fat dairy products, fat is not an issue. Plant protein is mainly found in nuts, legumes and, to a lesser extent, in vegetables.

Many people are confused about the amount of protein the body needs. The box on pages 28–29 gives specific amounts of food, but as a rule of thumb, you require a daily minimum of about 1 to 1.2 grams of pure protein

Text continued on page 30.

GOOD SOURCES OF PROTEIN

For the average person, the amounts of food given in this table constitute one palm; this provides the amount of protein we need for each of our three main meals. All of the amounts denote cooked and prepared food. The best choices are those that are lean, not processed (sausages, etc.) and not exposed to very high temperatures.

FISH AND SHELLFISH
Best choice

- All fish and shellfish - 3–4 ounces

Note: white fish and shellfish are low in fat. Oily fish—sardines, herring, mackerel, salmon, tuna, trout—are rich in omega-3 fatty acids (see page 36), so aim to eat them at least twice a week.

MEAT AND POULTRY
Best choice

- Lean beef - 3 ounces
- Venison - 3 ounces
- Turkey breast or leg, skinless - 3 ounces
- Rabbit - 3 ounces
- Chicken breast or leg, skinless - 3 ounces

Medium-good choice

- Minced beef, less than 10% fat - 3 ounces
- Lean pork - 3 ounces
- Duck breast, skinless - 3 ounces
- Veal, lean - 3 ounces
- Lamb, lean - 3 ounces
- Ham, lean - 3 ounces

Least-good choice

- Bacon - 2 rashers, 2½ ounces
- Lamb liver - 3 ounces
- Beef with fat - 3 ounces
- Chicken liver - 3 ounces
- Minced beef, more than 10% fat - 3 ounces
- Salami - 2 ounces
- Frankfurter (hot dog) - 2 sausages, 3½ ounces
- Pork sausages - 2, 2½ ounces

Note: liver is quite nutritious, but it is the "detox" organ of the body, so this meat is likely to contain toxins. If you like liver, I suggest that you serve calves' liver as a very occasional treat; the younger the animal, the fewer toxins should be in its liver.

EGGS

- 3 whole eggs
- 5 egg whites

Note: for most people this will be too many eggs. You could therefore combine, for example, two eggs with a smaller amount of another protein source. It has now been established that the cholesterol in eggs has no bearing on your blood cholesterol.

DAIRY PRODUCTS

Best choice

- Cottage cheese - 3 ounces
- Protein powder - 1 ounce

Medium-good choice

- Low-fat cheese, less than 10% fat - 3 ounces
- Ricotta - 3 ounces

Note: cheeses such as Cheddar, Brie, goat's cheese and Stilton may be eaten in small amounts as a snack, but always together with low-glycemic vegetables or low-glycemic fruit—not with medium- or high-glycemic carbohydrates such as bread or crackers. A matchbox-sized piece of cheese weighs about 1–1½ ounces and provides 6 to 8 grams of protein, but also lots of saturated fat.

MIXED PROTEIN AND CARBOHYDRATE SOURCES

Best choice

- Beans, lentils, chickpeas, tofu - 5 ounces
- Nonfat milk - 8 fluid ounces
- Buttermilk - 8 fluid ounces
- Yogurt, natural - 4 ounces

Medium-good choice

- Semi-skimmed milk, soy milk - 8 fluid ounces

Note: all unsweetened yogurt with live cultures is good because it replenishes healthy bacteria in your intestines. If you're trying to lose weight, choose fat-free or low-fat yogurt.

per 2 pounds of body weight (based on a "normal" healthy weight) if you are not particularly physically active. If you weigh 154 pounds, you will need a minimum of 70 to 84 grams of pure protein a day. And if you are physically active, whether at work or in sports, or are pregnant or breastfeeding, you will need more. Note that we are talking about pure protein here, not the amount of food: since meat, chicken, fish and certain nuts (almonds, cashews, peanuts) contain approximately 20 to 30 percent protein, you would need to eat 350 grams (about 12 ounces) of these foods to get 70 grams of pure protein.

Let me emphasize that this is not a high-protein diet. The amount of protein is somewhat higher than most of us are used to (at the expense of carbohydrates), but the total amount is not high. Protein itself is very satiating and it is difficult to overeat on protein alone—it's the bread or burger buns, potatoes and fries that go with it that cause many of today's health problems.

Protein—your fat-fighting friend

As well as providing the building blocks of our bodies, protein plays an important role in fighting body fat. It helps build calorie-burning muscle, but it also stimulates production of the growth hormone IGF-1 and a hormone called glucagon. The growth hormone increases muscle mass, while glucagon not only increases our sense of fullness after a meal, it also, most importantly, promotes the burning of body fat to provide energy. Glucagon's main function is to increase blood sugar if it is falling (for instance, during fasting or between meals), thus ensuring a steady energy supply for the body. Blood sugar is released from the liver's sugar supply (glycogen) and is also produced from proteins and fat. When the body is producing glucagon it is not producing insulin—which means less fat storage and more burning of body fat.

Carbohydrates

Carbohydrates are generally divided into two groups: sugars (simple carbohydrates) and starches (complex carbohydrates). Most people associate carbohydrates with bread, cereals, rice and pasta, while potatoes, apples and carrots, for example, are considered separately, as vegetables and fruit. But vegetables and fruit also contain carbohydrates, in addition to water, fiber (a non-digestible carbohydrate), vitamins and minerals. Sweet foods, such as sugar, honey, cookies and ice cream, are also carbohydrates.

Carbohydrates are not an essential part of the human diet in the same way proteins and some fats are because the body can produce all the carbohydrates it needs from proteins and fats. However, many foods containing carbohydrates also provide vitamins and minerals that are essential to good health. In addition, carbohydrate foods are the body's—and in particular the brain's—preferred source of energy. After they have been digested, more or less all carbohydrates end up in the blood as glucose—hence blood glucose, or blood sugar, as most people call it. Our brain is absolutely dependent on a stable supply of blood sugar, and it uses about 75 percent of all the glucose that circulates in our blood. This explains why a low blood sugar level, known as hypoglycemia, leads to considerable discomfort.

Healthy carbohydrates

Some foods lead to a gentle, low rise in blood sugar. They contain relatively few carbohydrates and a lot of fiber and water. These carbohydrates are slowly transformed into blood sugar in the body, and they do not particularly stimulate the production of insulin. This results in less fat storage and other undesirable consequences of a high blood sugar and insulin level. These foods should constitute the B part of the AB/C plate model, and they should always be combined with an appropriate amount of protein and unsaturated fat. The table on the opposite page gives a range of examples. Using the palm measurement, this will mean two palms of this kind of food when putting together an AB meal and about one and a half palms with the ABC reward meal.

EXAMPLES OF LOW-GLYCEMIC CARBOHYDRATES

RAW VEGETABLES

- Alfalfa sprouts
- Arugula
- Bamboo shoots
- Bok choy
- Broccoli
- Cabbage
- Carrots
- Cauliflower
- Celery, celery root
- Chicory
- Cucumber
- Endive
- Fennel
- Lettuce, all kinds
- Mushrooms, all kinds
- Onions, spring
  onions, leeks
- Peas
- Peppers
- Radishes
- Spinach
- Tomatoes
- Water chestnuts
- Watercress

COOKED VEGETABLES

- Artichokes (globe,
  Jerusalem)
- Asparagus
- Beans (fresh, dried,
  canned)
- Beets
- Broccoli
- Brussels sprouts
- Cabbage
- Carrots
- Cauliflower
- Celery root
- Chickpeas
- Eggplant
- Fennel
- Green beans
- Hummus (chickpea
  puree)
- Lentils (all kinds)
- Mushrooms
- Okra
- Onions, spring
  onions, leeks
- Peas
- Pumpkin
- Spinach
- Zucchini

FRUIT

- Apples
- Apricots
- Blackberries
- Black currants
- Blueberries
- Cherries
- Grapefruit
- Grapes
- Kiwi fruit
- Lemons, limes
- Melons
- Nectarines
- Oranges
- Peaches
- Pears
- Pineapple (fresh)
- Plums
- Red currants
- Strawberries
- Tangerines
- Watermelon

SWEET BUT DANGEROUS

Is there room for sweet things in a healthy diet? Of course there is. However, the source of sweetness you choose is very important. Sugars are part of the cellular structure of many foods, such as whole fruit and vegetables. It is not these but the vast amount of so-called added sugars—those found in honey, table sugar (and all other sugar types such as brown, cane, raw), fruit juices, baked goods, confectionery, convenience foods and so on—that are causing so many of today's health problems. If you wish to lose weight or gain control of your blood sugar levels, wherever possible you should avoid products that contain sucrose, or table sugar; glucose, glucose syrup or corn syrup (these concentrated syrups are widely used by the food industry); honey (which contains glucose, fructose and sucrose); and maltose, the kind of sugar that is found in beer.

As you are probably aware, the sugar contained in fruit is fructose. Fructose reacts differently in the body than other kinds of sugar. It is absorbed more slowly and cannot be converted into energy immediately. Fructose has a very small effect on blood sugar, and a medium GL of 19 (the GL of sucrose is 68). Wherever possible, you should substitute fructose or no-cal sweeteners for other sugars, but also reduce your consumption of sugar in all forms. Fruit is not recommended in unlimited quantities; in particular limit your intake of fruits such as bananas and mangoes, which have a higher GL than most other fruits. In general I recommend no more than two portions of fruit a day.

Less favorable carbohydrates

Some carbohydrates cause a quick rise in blood sugar and stimulate the pancreas to produce a lot of insulin. Unfortunately, many of our favorite foods (bread, potatoes, cake) fall into this category. By reducing the intake (both the amount and the frequency) of such foods, and by combining them with the right amount of protein and healthy, predominantly unsaturated fat and dietary fiber, we can avoid negative consequences to our health. You can allow yourself one meal a day that includes these foods—your reward meal. That will constitute the C part of the ABC plate model. If you use the palm measurement, that means half a palm of these foods a day. Use the tables at the back of the book to discover just how high-glycemic some of how your favorite carbohydrates are and try to choose those with the lowest GL. The higher the GL, the less you should eat.

Fats

Fat is our densest source of energy: It contains 9 calories per gram, whereas protein and carbohydrates contain 4 calories per gram. Despite its tarnished image, fat is a very important part of a healthy diet. Among other things, it is an important source of the fat-soluble vitamins A, D, E and K. However, as with protein and carbohydrates, you need to choose your source wisely.

All fatty foods contain both saturated and unsaturated fatty acids, but are usually described as either saturated or unsaturated, depending on the proportions of fatty acids present. Unsaturated fats can be further divided into monounsaturated and polyunsaturated. The human body is able to produce saturated and monounsaturated fatty acids, but not some types of polyunsaturated fatty acids. Some of these, however, are essential for good health; the only way we can obtain these is through our diet. These are called essential fatty acids, usually referred to as omega-3 and omega-6.

Choosing fats and oils

Monounsaturated fat: This should be the type of fat you eat most of, as monounsaturated fat provides good (HDL) cholesterol and helps keep down bad (LDL) cholesterol. Almonds, avocados, Brazil nuts, cashew nuts, hazelnuts, macadamia nuts, olives, peanuts, pecan nuts and pistachio nuts are very rich in monounsaturated fat. The healthiest types of oils are olive oil, canola oil and avocado oil, as these contain mainly monounsaturated fat. **Omega-3, polyunsaturated fat:** Most of us get too little omega-3 fatty acids and should increase our intake. Omega-3s have many benefits: in particular they have a protective effect against cardiovascular disease; and because they are an essential component of the brain, they are thought to lift

FATS AND OILS

The amounts given can be included in every meal. Athletes and people with physically demanding jobs should increase their intake of fat, mainly unsaturated fat.

BEST CHOICE

- Almonds, chopped - 4 tsp
- Almonds, cashew nuts, hazelnuts - 10–12
- Avocado - 3 tbs or ¼ to ½ of an avocado
- Brazil nuts - 2
- Canola oil, avocado oil, cold-pressed - 1 tsp
- Flaxseed, ground - 3–4 tsp
- Olive oil, extra virgin - 1 tsp
- Macadamia nuts - 3–5
- Olives - 8–10
- Natural peanut butter - 2 tsp
- Peanuts, pistachios - 18
- Pine nuts, pumpkin seeds, sunflower seeds - 2 tbs
- Walnuts - 6–8 halves

- Vinaigrette - 1 tsp olive oil and 2 tsp vinegar
- Sesame paste (tahini) - 2 tsp

MEDIUM-GOOD CHOICE

- Butter, ghee (clarified butter) - 1 tsp
- Mayonnaise - 1 tsp (preferably made with cold-pressed canola or olive oil)
- Sesame oil - 1.5 tsp (preferably cold-pressed)
- Single cream - 3 tbs

POORER CHOICE

(a lot of unsaturated fat or too much omega-6 fat)

- Whipping cream - 2 tbs
- Sour cream - 1 tbs
- Cream cheese - 3 tsp
- Low-fat cream cheese - 6 tsp
- Margarine - 1 tsp (but preferably do not use at all)
- Corn oil - 1 tsp (not suitable for frying)
- Soy bean oil - 1 tsp (not suitable for frying)

depression and even improve intelligence. The best source is oily fish such as salmon, sardines, mackerel, herring and tuna, as well as cod liver oil (as a supplement). Flaxseed is the richest source of omega-3 in the plant world, with as much as 58 percent health-friendly omega-3 fatty acids.

Omega-6, polyunsaturated fat: Though essential, omega-6 fatty acids are consumed in far greater quantities than necessary in the modern world. Corn, sunflower, safflower and soy bean oils, and the margarines derived from them, are all high in omega-6s and are widely used both in home cooking and by the food industry. To reduce your intake, switch from using sunflower, corn, soy and other refined oils and margarines to cold-pressed or extra-virgin oils—mainly olive oil and canola oil—and avoid eating fried foods too frequently.

Saturated fat: Many people eat far more saturated fat than they need: it is found in full-fat dairy products, meat, cake, cookies and pastries. Saturated fat is nonessential and thus not desirable in large quantities because it displaces the healthier and essential unsaturated fat. Moderate amounts of saturated fat will not do you any harm; it is when saturated fats are eaten to excess, as part of a high-glycemic diet, that problems arise.

Trans fats: These man-made fats, also known as hydrogenated (or partially hydrogenated) vegetable oils and fats, should be avoided wherever possible. Trans fatty acids are

FIBER

Although dietary fiber (an indigestible form of carbohydrate)
contributes very little energy, it plays a very important role in
human health. Almost all the fiber that we get from our diet comes
from vegetables, fruit, legumes, grains and nuts. There are two
main types of fiber: soluble and insoluble. Soluble fiber ensures the
proper digestion of nutrients, and means the bowels absorb
carbohydrates more slowly and thus blood sugar rises at a steadier
level over a longer period of time. Soluble fiber also lowers
cholesterol and is prebiotic (i.e., it supports good intestinal health).
Soluble fiber is found in beans and lentils, oats, vegetables and
fruit. Non-soluble dietary fiber, which is found in whole grains,
increases the volume of food and aids bowel function. It is also
believed that the fiber in our diet can prevent some forms of
cancer, such as colon cancer, but this might also be due to other
substances in fruit and vegetables.

Most people in the Western world consume less than 20 grams
of fiber daily. The official recommendation is 30 grams daily. An
easy way to increase your intake of dietary fiber is to eat two
pieces of fruit, at least three to four servings of vegetables a day
and plenty of lentils and beans (instead of potatoes and bread).
When you increase the amount of fiber in your diet, you should
also increase your water intake to ensure regular bowel function.

associated with a greatly increased risk of heart disease and many other inflammatory and degenerative diseases. They are found in many margarines and vegetable shortenings, and are widely used in the food industry. The majority of ready-made foods contain trans fats, so always check the labels and avoid foods that list "partially hydrogenated" fat or oil among the ingredients.

How much fat do you need?

Roughly one third of your total energy intake should derive from healthy, minimally processed fat. For an inactive person who weighs around 154 pounds, this means about 60–75 grams of fat a day, or the equivalent of 4–5 tablespoons. Divided among four to five meals a day, we are obviously talking about moderate amounts. Around 2 percent of this fat should derive from omega-3 fatty acids; 3 to 6 percent should derive from omega-6 fatty acids. Not more than 10 to 15 percent should derive from saturated fat and the rest, the biggest part, should come from monounsaturated fat.

The table on page 37 shows the total amount of fat you should eat with every meal to balance proteins and carbohydrates (when using the palm measurement) and highlights the sources of fat you should be enjoying and those that should be reduced or kept to a minimum.

A TYPICAL DAY WITH THE EASY GL DIET

BREAKFAST
- Scrambled eggs or an omelette made from 1 whole egg and 2 egg whites, chopped spinach and mushrooms fried with 1 teaspoon olive oil

SNACK
- 4½ ounces fat-free or low-fat natural yogurt with 3½ ounces fresh berries (optional: 1 teaspoon fructose or artificial sweetener)

LUNCH
- 3½–7 ounces grilled chicken breast or salmon (with herbs, spices, lemon, vinegar or mustard)
- mixed salad (e.g., 7 ounces salad leaves, tomato, red cabbage, cucumber, red onion, radish, 5 ounces cooked beans or lentils)
- salad dressing: 3 teaspoons olive oil with 1 to 3 teaspoons balsamic vinegar or lemon juice, ½ teaspoon Dijon mustard or herbs (optional)

SNACK
(could be eaten after dinner, if dinner is early)
- 1 pear
- 10 whole almonds

DINNER
- about a cup of pea soup or lentil soup
- 4–5 ounces grilled or steamed salmon (with herbs, spices)
- 7 ounces steamed broccoli with 1 teaspoon olive oil
- 3½ ounces boiled basmati rice or spaghetti

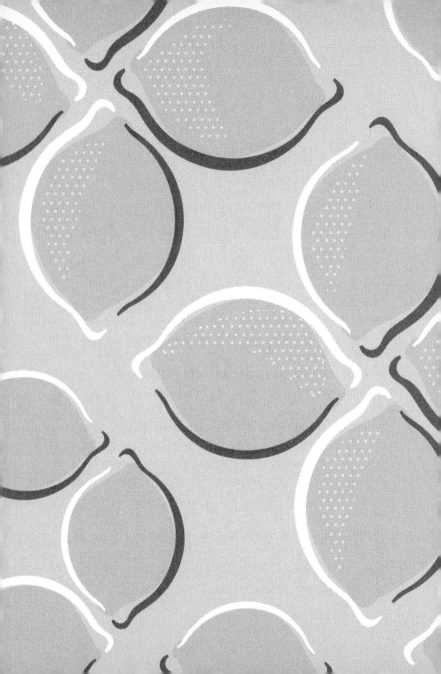

Shopping:
Make The Right Choices

If you want to follow the principles of a low-glycemic diet, the obvious starting point is to choose the correct foods with which to stock your kitchen. Many of us do our food shopping on auto-pilot, buying the same foods week after week—regardless of their negative effect on our health. This chapter will help refresh your shopping habits and set you on the path to improved blood sugar control and better all-around health.

Before we look at specific foods, I want to make a general—but very important—point: the human body needs natural whole foods. As much as possible that means foods that do not have a label—for example, vegetables, fruit, nuts, fish and meat—or those that have been minimally processed, such as cold-pressed (extra-virgin) oils and natural dairy produce, especially unsweetened yogurt and fresh cheeses such as cottage cheese and fromage frais. If your shopping cart contains lots of products with long lists of ingredients then you will not become truly healthy. Of course we all indulge in a treat now and again, but the bulk of our diets should be made up of the foods that nature intended for us.

Vegetables

When it comes to natural whole foods, vegetables reign supreme. They are crucial to your health and aid weight reduction. Because of the soluble fiber in vegetables, the carbohydrates are absorbed slowly, gradually converting to blood sugar. This leads to a lower and more stable insulin level in the blood. The non-soluble fiber in vegetables increases the volume of food and the feeling of satiety. Most vegetables are low GL and you'll find an extensive list of appropriate choices—both raw and cooked—on page 33.

It is important to eat a wide variety of vegetables but it also makes sense to buy those that are in season locally, as they tend to have the best flavor and the lowest price.

Some vegetables have a medium GL—for example, sweet potatoes, yams and corn—but you do not need to avoid these, simply eat them in moderation.

Fresh vegetables offer a marvelous range of flavors and textures, but do not forget frozen vegetables—they are a valuable source of nutrients and in fact often retain more of their natural vitamins. Peas, leaf spinach, green beans and broccoli freeze well.

Some canned vegetables are also useful: no kitchen should be without canned tomatoes, while more unusual vegetables such as artichoke hearts are convenient and taste great with olive oil, garlic and lemon juice.

One other must-have in the kitchen is avocado. You won't find it on the list of low-glycemic vegetables because it contains more fat than carbohydrate, but it is a very good source of healthy fats. I use it in soups, as well as dips and salads.

Fruit

Fruit is very important to a balanced diet as it is a good source of vitamins, minerals and other antioxidants. Many types of fruit have a low GL because they are high in fiber and because fructose, the sugar found in fruit, has a low GI. On page 33 you'll find a list of low-glycemic fruits. Don't just stick to old favorites. As with vegetables, choose whatever is in season first and foremost because it will be tastier and have better value. Canned fruit (as long

LEMONS AND LIMES

Research shows that acid in food (for example, lemon and other citrus fruits, vinegar) reduces the glycemic effect of the meal.

Make sure that lemons and limes are on your shopping list every week. Look for unwaxed and preferably organic fruit—that way the grated zest will taste of fruit rather than waxy chemicals! Use lemon and lime juice:

- in salad dressings
- with fish, chicken and meat
- with grilled and roasted vegetables
- in savory and sweet sauces
- in fruit salads

as it is in unsweetened juice) and frozen fruit can be a useful standby, and frozen berries in particular are great for making smoothies.

A few fresh fruits, for instance bananas, have a medium GL so you should not eat them quite as often as low-GL fruits. Most dried fruits have a very high GL and should be avoided, though occasional small amounts eaten with low-GL fruits and protein foods (e.g., yogurt) are acceptable.

Legumes

Not just for vegetarians—beans, lentils and chickpeas are a staple of healthy traditional diets around the world. Supermarkets and smaller shops offer a huge choice, both dried and canned: red kidney beans, white haricot beans, black beans, pinto beans, mung beans ... Generally, beans and legumes have a low GL and provide protein as well as healthy carbohydrate, fiber, vitamins, minerals and healthy fatty acids. Soy beans are higher in protein and fat and lower in carbohydrates than other beans but they are not as widely available. If you want more stable blood sugar, the answer is simple: Eat more beans and legumes!

Dried beans and chickpeas that have been soaked and cooked have a slightly lower GL than their canned counterparts but the difference is not significant. Dried beans have a slightly better taste and firmer texture, but canned beans are more convenient to use. If you do soak your own beans—it's not difficult, you just need to plan ahead—it is a good idea to cook a big portion. They will keep for days in the fridge and for as long as six months in the freezer. Frozen broad beans are an inexpensive and very versatile ingredient.

Dried lentils do not need to be soaked, but they do need to be boiled for 20 to 30 minutes. If you are new to lentils try red lentils or dark green Puy lentils, both of which have a lovely flavor. Canned lentils are also widely available; they tend to sink to the bottom of the can so shake well before opening.

Grains
Bread
Buying bread often makes us feel a bit like a child in a candy store—there is so much to choose from and it all looks so tempting, even though we know it is not necessarily good for us. Just how healthy is bread for you? It varies significantly, depending on the type of flour it is made from. The finer the flour, the quicker blood sugar and insulin will rise after it is eaten. The GL of bread per 100 grams varies between 30 and 50. Fine flour gives a quicker and higher rise in blood sugar than sugar—something few people realize. Unfortunately, most of the bread that is sold contains more than 80 percent fine wheat flour, which gives you a lot of energy, but little nourishment.

When buying bread do not be fooled by products described as "brown" or "multi-grain" bread. They generally contain mostly fine wheat flour because it is the cheapest raw material there is. The color of a bread does not necessarily indicate that it is a whole-grain product—if you use sufficient color (malt), you could make fine bread that is almost black. And a bread that is "multi-grain" need not contain any "whole" grains at all. What matters is how coarse and heavy the bread is. Whole grains weigh more than fine flour, and this is how you can assess how coarse a loaf of bread is. The coarser the bread, the lower the GL.

The type of grain is also important. Rye and barley give a lower GL than wheat. However, if you prefer wheat breads, look for a heavy loaf that is labeled "stone-ground whole grain." Alternatively, you may be able to find bread made from spelt. Spelt is an ancient type of wheat that has become increasingly popular in recent years. It has roughly the same GL as whole-grain wheat (i.e., relatively high, but it contains a bit more protein, more fiber and more vitamins and minerals). It also seems to be tolerated better than wheat by those with poor tolerance to regular wheat.

Nuts and seeds such as sunflower, sesame, flaxseed and pumpkin will also reduce the GI of bread and at the same time add more protein, healthy fat and fiber. Sourdough bread also has a somewhat lower GL because acidity reduces the glycemic effect of foods.

SNACKS

Our metabolism becomes more efficient the more frequently we eat. Aim to eat every three to four hours: three main meals and two snacks in between. Skipping a meal or snack will slow your metabolism. For each snack, choose one item from the protein column and one from the carbohydrates.

PROTEIN

- 3½–5 ounces cottage cheese or fromage frais
- 3½–4½ ounces natural yogurt
- 1 tablespoon pumpkin, sunflower or sesame seeds
- 8–10 almonds
- 2–4 Brazil nuts
- 10–12 cashew nuts
- 8–10 hazelnuts
- 4–6 macadamia nuts
- 12–18 peanuts
- 2–3 teaspoons natural, unsweetened peanut butter
- 4–8 walnuts or pecans
- 2 tablespoons hummus
- 3 ounces prawns, smoked salmon or tuna

CARBOHYDRATE

- unlimited raw vegetables, such as: bean sprouts, carrots, cauliflower, celery, chicory, cucumber, fennel, lettuce, mushrooms, peppers, spinach, tomatoes, watercress, zucchini
- 3½ ounces fresh berries
- 3½ ounces grapes
- 1 peach or nectarine
- 1 apple
- 1 pear
- 1 orange or 2 satsumas
- 1 kiwi fruit
- 3 fresh or dried apricots
- 1 slice watermelon
- ½ small melon
- 8 olives
- 1–1½ ounces plain dark chocolate (70% cocoa solids)

Coarse bread is more expensive than bread made from highly refined flour, but remember that you pay a lot for air when you buy baguettes. Keep in mind, though, that even the coarsest bread will range from medium to high GL—it is never low GL.

Look for: 100 percent stone-ground whole grain

Crispbread

There is a wide selection of crispbread, but it is difficult to know the GL of these products because few of them have been tested. When selecting crispbread, the type of grain and the fiber content are very important. Varieties that contain rye are often a good choice since rye has a lower GI than wheat. However, do not simply assume that a rye crispbread is a healthier choice—check that the fiber content is high, too. The higher the fiber content, the lower the GL. Health food shops are more likely than supermarkets to stock high-fiber crispbreads—for example, some Scandinavian crispbreads contain as much as 85 percent unprocessed bran.

Pasta

Many people are surprised to learn that pasta has a lower GI than bread. That is because pasta normally is made from durum wheat (semolina), which has a lower GI than regular wheat. Durum wheat flour is coarser and contains somewhat more protein. And remember, the less you cook the pasta, the lower its GL. Pasta *al dente*, which gives you something to chew on, is better for the blood sugar than pasta that has cooked for longer.

When shopping for pasta, opt for one made from whole-grain durum wheat since it contains more fiber, vitamins and minerals than regular "white" pasta. It was once only available in health food shops but most supermarkets now sell it either in the form of spaghetti or fusilli. If you are lucky, you will also find protein-enriched pasta, where 20 to 30 percent soy protein has been added to the pasta.

Pasta can also be made by partially using other types of flour, such as barley, flour from white lentils, mung beans and soy beans, which give a much lower GI. On the other hand, gluten-free pasta is normally made from corn, millet or buckwheat, which gives it a higher GL.

Best options: whole-wheat spaghetti, protein-enriched pasta, mung bean pasta (cellophane or glass noodles)

Rice

There is a wide—and confusing—array of rice varieties out there, but which of them is best for your blood sugar? Rice can vary from medium to high GI, depending on type and how it is cooked. Short-grained, sticky Asian (jasmine and sushi) rice has a high GL and should be avoided. Long-grain basmati rice is a better choice. "Parboiled" long-grain American rice also has a lower GL than sticky rice since it is steamed before being processed further, making it less sticky. As a rule of thumb: the stickier the rice after it has been cooked, the higher the GL.

Brown rice does not have a significantly lower GI than parboiled white rice but it does contain more of the outer husk and is richer in fiber, vitamins and minerals, so it is the healthiest choice. Wild rice, which is not a rice but a grass plant, is another good choice because it has a low GI, lots of fiber and a pleasant nutty taste. It is expensive but can be mixed with other kinds of rice.

Best options: brown basmati, wild rice

Oats

Oats have a low GL—but I'm referring to old-fashioned rolled oats (the ones with the big flakes), not the pre-cooked "instant" variety, which have a higher GL. You can use oats to make porridge, of course, but oatmeal can also replace some of the wheat flour in many recipes, such as muffins, bread, pancakes, biscuits, pie pastry and pizzas.

Oat bran has a relatively low GL and a gently sweet taste so it reduces the need for sugar in recipes. The high content of soluble fiber can also reduce the need for fat. You can replace as much as 25 to 50 percent of the wheat flour with oat bran in recipes such as muffins, cakes, pancakes and cookies.

Other useful grains

Barley: Barley has a pleasantly nutty taste and a low GL. It can be an excellent alternative to rice and potatoes, as a side dish or in soups and stews. You can also use it when you bake, but remember that barley contains very little gluten so if you want bread that leavens and is elastic, you need to add 10 grams of gluten flour per 100 grams of barley flour. Gluten flour is available from health food shops.

Buckwheat: Roasted buckwheat kernels (also called "kasha") have a low–medium GL of 11 and are a good alternative to rice, pasta and potatoes. If your supermarket doesn't sell buckwheat, you should be able to find it in a health food shop.

Bulgur and couscous: Bulgur is coarsely chopped durum wheat that has been partially pre-cooked and dried; couscous is simply a finer variety of bulgur. Both take just a few minutes to prepare and are a good choice of grain, having a GL of 7 to 8. Couscous and bulgur are widely available in supermarkets.

Quinoa: Called the "mother grain" by the Incas, quinoa is high in protein and has a low GL. It has a slightly nutty flavor and is a good alternative to rice in savory dishes. It is widely available in health food shops and larger supermarkets.

Breakfast cereals

Breakfast cereals are easy and convenient; many people eat them every day. If you are one of those people, it is important to find a cereal that is minimally processed and unsweet-ened. This can be tricky, as supermarket shelves are groan-ing under the weight of unhealthy high-GL cereals, mostly prepared from highly processed grains. Corn flakes, for example, have a very high GL. Did you know that a 30-gram serving of corn flakes gives you an increase in blood sugar and insulin similar to an equal amount of pure sugar?

When shopping for cereals look for those that are high in fiber—All-Bran is a good example—and have no added sugar. Don't assume that because something has a "healthy" reputation it will be suitable for a low-glycemic lifestyle—muesli is often sweetened and most brands contain dried fruit, which has a high GL. A much better alternative is unsweetened muesli made from grains and seeds, and with a minimal amount of dried fruit (preferably none at all).

Whichever cereal you choose, if you add milk and berries, chopped nuts, ground flaxseeds or soy flakes, or a spoonful of yogurt, this will lower its GL. And if you must sweeten your cereal, use a little fructose.

Look for: unsweetened, whole-wheat or whole-grain cereals

Sugars

While I recommend that you reduce your consumption of sugars, most people are unlikely to eat none at all—so what are the best options? Avoid sucrose (i.e., table sugar, glucose, honey, corn syrup, molasses and golden syrup). Fructose,

BREAKFASTS

A good breakfast is vital to kick-start your metabolism in the morning and provide energy to get you through the first part of the day. Do not make the common mistake of having a breakfast that consists mainly of carbohydrates. Breakfast should be considered a main meal like any other and should always include a palm-sized serving of protein. Protein enhances the body's ability to burn fat and satisfies your appetite far better than carbohydrates alone.

Think beyond whole-grain cereals and try featuring some of the following in your breakfast repertoire:

- Cottage cheese
- Eggs
- Grilled, lean Canadian bacon
- Natural unsweetened yogurt or soy yogurt
- Nuts and seeds
- Peanut butter
- Salmon
- Smoothies enriched with protein powder

Breakfast is also a good time to have a portion of fruit or vegetables, so have some unsweetened fruit juice, berries on your oats, or tomatoes, mushrooms or spinach with your scrambled eggs or omelette.

which is the type of sugar contained in fruit, is a much better option, with a GL of 19—compared to sucrose's GL of 68. Fructose is sold in granular form in health food shops and supermarkets, but it is more expensive to produce than sucrose—which is why it is not widely used in food manufacturing. However, it is 30 to 50 percent sweeter than ordinary sugar, so you need less to obtain the same level of sweetness. (It also provides 30 to 50 percent fewer calories than ordinary sugar). Limit your fructose intake to a maximum of 30 to 50 grams per day: remember that fructose is not a necessary part of a healthy diet, it is just a better alternative to ordinary sugar when you want to prepare a dessert or cake.

Artificial sweeteners such as aspartame, saccharin, acesulfame-K and sucralose (Splenda) cause a small, almost insignificant, rise in blood sugar, and are an acceptable alternative to sugar, when eaten in moderation.

Oils and fats

Many people are confused about the best type of oils to use in the kitchen. On page 36 I outlined the sorts of fats that are essential, those that can be eaten in moderation and those that should be avoided. What does this advice mean when you are standing in front of row upon row of oils? Quite simply, look for oils labeled "virgin" or "cold-pressed," which means they are as natural as possible and have not been refined using heat or chemicals. Extra-virgin olive oil and cold-pressed canola, sesame, walnut and avocado oils are all readily available. These oils are suitable for a variety of uses: extra-virgin olive oil has a lovely flavor and is good for everyday use; the neutral taste of canola oil is good when you want to avoid the flavor of olives; sesame oil is great for Chinese food; and the more unusual (and expensive) cold-pressed nut and seed oils are delicious sprinkled over salads. One of my favorite oils is cold-pressed flaxseed oil. It is very rich in omega-3 fatty acids but should be used in small quantities to enrich your diet, not as your main source of fat.

Generally, oils that are not marked "cold-pressed" or "virgin" are highly processed to extend their shelf lives and are detrimental to health. This group includes corn, sunflower, safflower and vegetable oils.

Fats are also the subject of much confusion. A small amount of butter will be far less harmful to long-term health than frequent use of the highly processed margarines and spreads made from hydrogenated or partially hydrogenated fats—as these often contain trans fats. If you have to fry at high temperatures, use clarified butter (ghee) together with olive oil, canola oil or pure coconut oil. Butter ghee—not the vegetable (hardened) ghee substitute—tolerates higher temperatures.

Avoid: processed vegetable oils and any product that contains hydrogenated or partially hydrogenated fats

Proteins

Protein has no effect on blood sugar levels, so food that consists mainly of protein does not have a GI value. However, your choice of protein—and how it is cooked—can have a positive or negative effect on your health and make an important contribution to the benefits of following a Mediterranean-style diet.

Fish and shellfish

If you are searching for a source of healthy protein, start with fish and shellfish. As well as protein, they provide a multitude of vitamins and minerals. White fish such as sole and cod are very low in fat, while oily fish such as sardines and mackerel are high in beneficial omega-3 fats. All fish and shellfish are good for you, so don't get stuck in a rut: yes, salmon is tasty and readily available, but what about other oily fish such as trout and tuna? The only downside with larger oily fish such as tuna and swordfish is that they eat smaller fish and live longer, so they are more likely to accumulate toxins such as mercury; smaller fish are less likely to be contaminated to the same extent. The concerns about toxins in fish mean that we are now being advised to limit our intake of oily fish to three times a week. Pregnant women are advised to avoid oily fish but to eat plenty of white fish and to get their omega-3 fatty acids from high-quality supplements.

When buying fresh fish, look for bright eyes, red gills, a nice sheen or color and a plump or firm appearance.

Shellfish such as prawns, langoustines, scallops, squid, mussels and clams are quick to cook. However, they must be very fresh when you cook them: Sniff before you buy— you want a sea-fresh smell, not a fishy odor. At one time some shellfish were thought to raise cholesterol levels but scientists have now rejected this theory.

Canned seafood is a healthy choice; it is also convenient and good value. Opt for varieties canned in olive oil or spring water, rather than those in sunflower or other vegetable oil.

Chicken and other poultry

Chicken, turkey and other poultry are excellent sources of protein. One of the great advantages of poultry is that most of the fat, between 50 and 85 percent, is in the skin; which is easy to remove. The meat itself is fairly lean. Poultry contains quite a lot of B vitamins and is also rich in zinc, magnesium and iron.

When shopping for poultry, don't forget duck—it contains more iron than beef, and increased farming of the birds means that whole ducks and duck breasts are now commonplace in supermarkets. Be careful to cut all the fat off duck as some tends to cling to the meat after the skin has been removed.

Pork, bacon, ham and veal

If you choose lean cuts and trim off any visible fat, pork and veal are good sources of protein and also provide B vitamins and considerable amounts of minerals like potassium and zinc. When buying pork and veal, opt for tenderloin (often called fillet), medallions, escalopes or other cuts where any fat can easily be trimmed off.

If you like bacon, choose Canadian bacon rather than the streaky, trim-off-the-fat-before-cooking kind, and enjoy it as an occasional treat rather than every day. Lean ham is good for salads and lunches and it's easy to trim off the fat.

Beef and lamb

I do not eat red meat often because I prefer fish, chicken and turkey, but this does not mean that I never eat red meat. When I do, I choose the best and leanest cuts, such as fillet and rump steak, and trim off any fat. As an alternative to beef, ostrich is very low in fat and is becoming more widely available now that it is being farmed.

When I need ground meat, I always pick inexpensive pieces of meat with no fat and have the butcher mince it for me. It is also easy to do this using a food processor. This way you can be sure that the meat is lean. Pre-packed ground meat can contain a lot of fat (as well as ice water that you pay a high price for). Ground beef with less than 10 percent fat, available from some supermarkets, is the next best choice.

Game

Game is some of the healthiest meat you can eat. It is low in fat and high in iron. Game meat contains less fat between the muscle cells. The fat also contains a somewhat higher level of omega-3 fatty acids than regular red meat.

Now that venison is farmed it has become more popular and more widely available (at a price that most people can afford). Hare and wild rabbit are also good choices, though they are not very common anywhere other than at specialized butcher shops. Young game birds (for example, pheasant, partridge and wild duck) are quick to roast, while older birds make good casseroles; most are sold only during the winter season.

Eggs

Eggs are a valuable source of protein, and eggs from poultry that live in a free and natural way are a rich source of other nutrients. Your best option is to buy free-range eggs from a small farm. If this isn't possible, opt for free-range eggs from a shop with a high turnover (to ensure freshness).

Some shops now sell omega-3 eggs. These are from hens whose diet is supplemented with flaxseed or marine algae. Opt for the "vegetarian" eggs, as those from hens fed on marine algae or fishmeal sometimes have a slightly fishy, cod liver oil taste.

COOKING TIPS

- Frying, particularly deep frying, destroys the healthy unsaturated fatty acids in oils and causes the formation of toxic byproducts, including trans fatty acids. Roasting, steaming and grilling are preferable, particularly for fish and meat.

- If you are cooking meat with a low fat content (such as turkey), it is important to use low temperatures in order to retain the natural juices in the meat: this avoids the need for rich sauces. When cooking meat and poultry in the oven, it is best to use a meat thermometer or core temperature thermometer.

- Marinating meat in a mixture of lemon juice and olive oil before you cook it is a good idea; it is an excellent way to get a succulent result.

- When preparing a meat sauce with ground meat, you should gently heat the meat in a non-stick pan, without any fat, and then drain off the fat while it is still hot. You may very well add more healthy fat like olive oil afterwards.

- Avoid boiling vegetables since this leaches out water-soluble vitamins and trace minerals, which are then discarded along with the water. Steaming is a much better way to cook vegetables: vitamins and minerals are retained and the texture and flavor are superior.

- Never overcook vegetables—the more "bite" they have the greater their nutritional value.

Dairy products

Dairy products, though not essential for good health, are a source of high-quality protein and several vitamins and minerals, including calcium. Unfortunately, some are high in saturated fat. Your best choices of dairy proteins are natural yogurt and cottage cheese—both of which are an important part of my diet.

On the whole, you should avoid high-fat cheeses, though I do not recommend that you eat processed reduced-fat cheeses instead. If you are a cheese-lover, enjoy an occasional piece of high-fat cheese as a treat, and serve it with fruit or salad, as they do in France. I use small amounts of feta and Parmesan in salads and cooked vegetable dishes: with these strongly flavored cheeses, a little goes a long way.

I am not a great fan of milk—it contains a significant amount of the sugar lactose and, being a liquid, does not offer the same level of satiety as solid dairy foods. If you like milk, choose nonfat milk or low-fat, or try soy milk, which is a good alternative.

Avoid: cream, ice cream, yogurts with added sugar

Soy products

Soy is a good source of protein for everybody, but especially for vegetarians.

Soy beans have the highest protein content of all beans, are low GL and have many health-promoting qualities. Fresh soy beans (known as edamame) are not readily available unless you live near an Asian market, but there are many soy-based products. Opt for more natural products such as tofu, tempeh and soy milk rather than soy-based meat substitutes and cheeses, which are often highly processed.

Nuts and seeds

Nuts and seeds are a good source of protein and other nutrients, but are also high in fat, which is why they are listed under fats and oils on page 36. I recommend that you eat small amounts of nuts and seeds on a regular basis. Choose fresh, raw nuts and seeds, not roasted and salted, and do not store them for too long or the fats will turn rancid; they will keep longer if you store them in the freezer. Almonds, Brazil nuts, cashews, hazelnuts, peanuts, pine nuts, pistachios and walnuts are all good choices for snacks or to boost the protein content and reduce the glycemic load of your meals.

Peanut butter can be a healthy addition to your cupboard, as long as you choose a natural version with no added sugar. Other nut butters such as almond and cashew are becoming more widely available.

WHAT TO DRINK

Water is without doubt the best refreshment for the body and you should aim to drink at least 8 glasses a day. If you buy mineral water, look for a low-sodium brand, as some carbonated water is high in salt (sodium).

The following drinks contain a high amount of carbohydrates and should be avoided: all canned and bottled drinks containing sugar (including ready-made iced tea), most beers and lagers (opt for low-carb beer if available), sweet wines, liqueurs. Also avoid fizzy drinks containing artificial sugars (these are thought to damage teeth and promote osteoporosis). Milk is often thought of as a healthy drink because of its calcium content, but it also contains a significant amount of sugar in the form of lactose so it is best drunk in moderation (there are plenty of other healthy sources of calcium, including figs, tofu, beans, spinach and broccoli). Coffee should also be consumed in moderation, as large amounts can be detrimental to health. Tea has been shown to have a number of health benefits; however, green tea is preferable to black, which does not have the wide range of benefits of green tea.

A glass of wine—especially red—with a meal has been found to have a number of health benefits, but if you are trying to lose weight I recommend that you avoid all alcohol for a few weeks.

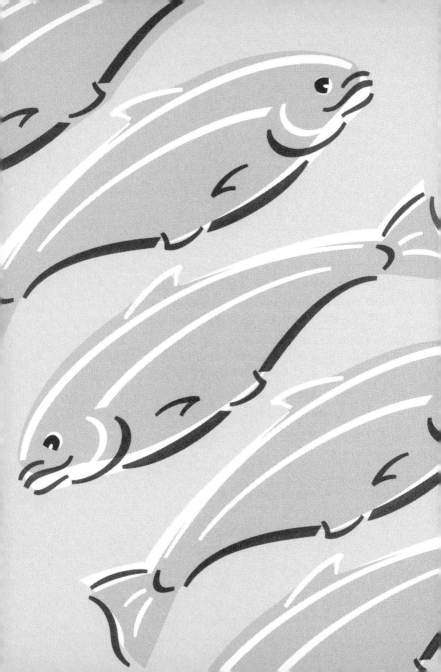

Eating Out:
How to Stay on Track

Eating out is one of the great pleasures of life and is some-thing that many people now do on a very regular basis. Let's face it, a busy, hectic lifestyle doesn't always allow us to cook our own food. But when you cook for your-self, you are in charge of your diet and its effect on your health; when eating out, you allow others to influence your diet and health.

Unfortunately, the food industry's motivations and goals are often incompatible with those of someone following a healthy diet. This is particularly true of the fast-food indus-try, which has focused on producing and offering foods that are safe in terms of hygiene, quick to prepare and consume, inexpensive and widely available. But they are seldom healthy. Quality costs money and food is no exception. You expect to pay more for a better TV or car—why should food be different? I am not saying you should not be price-conscious, but in the case of food, the long-term result of focusing on low price alone is poor health.

Thankfully, once you move away from the fast-food out-lets, the trend towards healthier foods is evident in many restaurants and bars. Eating out and eating healthily is absolutely possible. In fact it is easy. I will try to help you along the way, so that you can make wise, healthy choices without becoming obsessed or feeling deprived.

Always remember that YOU are the customer, and that any quality restaurant should walk the extra mile to please you. Don't be shy—ask the waiter if you could have more vegetables or legumes in exchange for fries, or the dressing or sauce of your choice served on the side.

General recommendations

- Don't arrive at the restaurant extremely hungry. You will be able to make far wiser choices from the menu if you have a small, low-glycemic, high-protein, high-fiber snack before leaving home. A small handful of nuts and a small portion of fruit or vegetables is perfect. A small bowl of All-Bran with unsweetened yogurt and some berries or pieces of fruit is another alternative. Make sure you drink a large glass of water with your snack or have one as soon as you arrive at the restaurant.
- Say no to the ubiquitous bread rolls that are passed around and ask the waiter not to leave the bread basket on the table to tempt you. Starting a meal with high-glycemic bread will increase your blood sugar and insulin, and even—temporarily—your appetite. Besides, why fill up with the inexpensive and unhealthier stuff at the risk

of not being able to finish off your main meal? If you wish, ask for vegetable crudités instead—carrot and celery sticks are a good, simple option that any restaurant should be able to provide.

- If possible, start your meal with a salad dressed with vinaigrette (olive oil and vinegar, or olive oil and lemon juice), as this will actually lower the glycemic load of the rest of the meal. This is because acidic foods such as vinegar and lemon juice delay the emptying of the stomach and therefore also the absorption of carbohydrates in the intestine; fat (oil) also slows down carbohydrate absorption. Make sure you ask for the dressing to be served separately, so that you can decide how much you use.

- If you choose a soup, opt for one based on stock (chunks of vegetable or legumes are OK) rather than a thick, creamy one.

- When considering the menu, try to visualize how your dinner plate should look in order to conform to the guide on pages 25 and 26. Are you having your ABC reward meal or a regular AB meal? If it's the latter, you may want to forego the rice, pasta or potatoes and opt for a double portion of vegetables, or ask if lentils, beans or chickpeas are available as an alternative. If this is your ABC meal, decide if you want the C part of the meal to be potatoes, rice or pasta, or if you would rather double the veggies and opt for a dessert instead.

- If you wish to eat meat, as a rule of thumb opt for poultry or lean cuts of red meat.
- Fish and shellfish are usually very good choices when eating out. Oily-fleshed fish (such as salmon, mackerel, tuna and trout) is an even healthier option than white fish and shellfish. Fried fish in batter or breadcrumbs is not such a good idea.
- Avoid any food that is battered or breadcrumbed and deep or shallow-fried.
- Remember that a dessert based on dairy products, eggs and/or nuts is better for you than one made with flour.

Bars

Once a haven of unhealthy food, bars have come a long way in recent years, due in part to the rise in popularity of simple high-quality foods and the growth of micro-breweries. However, the quality of food available is still very much dependent on location and the amount of competition there is. If you live in a large town or city, it is far easier to eat a healthy meal in a bar. Often the best healthy dishes will be those made from traditional ingredients but with a Mediterranean or Asian influence. The key to eating well in a bar is to keep it simple: opt for the high-quality sources of protein that are served with simple sauces and vegetables or salad. Avoid high-glycemic starters such as garlic bread, cheese-topped bruschetta and potato wedges;

for the main course steer clear of traditional fare such as hamburgers, baked or mashed potato, breaded and battered dishes, dishes loaded with gravy, butter and cheese. As far as desserts are concerned, bars and microbreweries are a dietary minefield—they seem to specialize in hugely fattening, high-GI/GL treats.

Best options:
Leaf salads without creamy dressings, vegetable-based dips with crudités, steamed mussels, grilled or baked fish and seafood, grilled steak or pork (lean cuts), game, steamed vegetables or vegetables roasted in olive oil

Avoid:
Rolls, garlic bread, bruschetta, croutons, nachos, creamy soups, Caesar salad, deep-fried or crumbed fish and seafood, fishcakes, vegetables in batter, mashed potatoes, burgers, french fries

Chinese

Traditional Chinese cuisine is one of the most delicious and varied in the world. Sadly, the quality of many Chinese take-out joints and restaurants does not reflect this rich heritage. Stir-frying should be a healthy way of cooking, but a lot of Chinese food is battered and then deep-fried in fat of dubious quality, and the end result is a dish that contains not only white flour and lots of fat, but unhealthy fat to boot. Pancake (spring) rolls are the perfect example

COPING WITH BUFFETS

All-you-can-eat buffets are not a good idea. The eye is almost always hungrier than the stomach and it is much easier to give in to temptation when everything lies presented beautifully before you. It is a fact that most people end up eating more from a buffet than if they have a three-course meal presented to them. And if you need to eat your buffet meal while standing, the effect is even worse: not only is there a tendency to overload one's plate, but the whole process of eating is much shorter. Satiety signals usually take 20 minutes to reach the brain, which makes it easily possible to overeat from a buffet or a fast-food outlet. Eating at a restaurant, where you have to wait between courses, allows you to feel satiated, even with smaller quantities. I often wonder how I could ever be satisfied with the small portions presented in gourmet restaurants, but I always am.

If choosing from a buffet is your only option, then following some basic rules may help you avoid the worst pitfalls.

Before putting anything on your plate, take a good look at everything that is available at the buffet. Then decide what you like best. Start by filling two-thirds of your dinner plate with vegetables and legumes, and then proceed to choose fish, seafood, poultry or meat. Once you've eaten that, allow at least 10 to 15 minutes before you return for seconds, and follow the same rule again. If you've decided to skip dessert, don't even bother to look at what's available or you'll probably give in to temptation.

of this. If you opt for dim sum and the method of cooking is not obvious, ask for steamed dim sum over anything fried.

Most Chinese restaurants use large quantities of sticky rice and noodles topped with stir-fried vegetables and meat, fish or poultry. The glutinous, short-grain rice used is very high GI and nutrient poor. More upmarket Chinese restaurants should offer the option of brown rice. Either way, limit the amount of rice you eat or skip it altogether. Noodles are usually made of wheat or rice and are equally problematic. Cellophane noodles, the ones made from mung beans, are a good alternative, if they are available. Always avoid fried crispy noodles.

Opt for stir-fried vegetables and grilled, baked or stir-fried (not deep-fried) chicken, beef, fish or shellfish in savory (not sweet), non-thickened sauces. Tofu is a very healthy meat alternative and is a good choice as long as it is not served in a sweet or thickened sauce. Unfortunately, many Chinese restaurants use flavor enhancers such as monosodium glutamate (MSG). Savory condiments and sauces like soy sauce and oyster sauce are high in sodium, but more upmarket restaurants will sometimes offer reduced-sodium (light) alternatives. One plus point is that Chinese food is usually rich in healthy antioxidant-rich spices, as well as garlic and ginger.

Best options:
Chicken mushroom soup; hot and sour soup; grilled satay dishes; steamed tofu; steamed fish with ginger; stir-fried poultry, meat or seafood with garlic and ginger or reduced-sodium soy or oyster sauce; steamed vegetables; cellophane (mung bean) noodles

Avoid:
Won ton soup, noodle soup, spring or pancake rolls, shrimp chips, dumplings, sweet and sour dishes, crispy duck, chow mein, rice

French restaurants/bistro style

France is one of the slimmest nations in the industrialized world, despite the country's high consumption of butter and cream. The key reasons for this are that the French have a tremendously varied diet and a high consumption of vegetables; they also display an admirable resistance to American-style fast food (although sadly that is beginning to change). It should be fairly easy to choose wisely at a French restaurant. Opt for a salad or a clear soup for a starter. There's usually a good choice of healthy, simply cooked (grilled, baked or steamed) main courses: steaks, lamb, chicken, duck, fish and shellfish, accompanied by various vegetables. Lentils (especially French Puy lentils) and beans are a great alternative to potatoes, rice or pasta as a side dish. Purées of vegetables like celery root and spinach can be healthy, as long as they are not laden with butter or cream. Try to avoid creamy sauces and soups, french fries and other potato dishes, crêpes and pastries. Opt for a fruit or berry dessert or—if you are having an ABC reward meal—a small, rich chocolate mousse, or small quantities of cheese with salad (not crackers or bread).

Best options:

Non-creamy vegetable soup, crudités, steamed mussels, leaf salad with poultry or seafood (with dressing on the side), meat or fish grilled with olive oil, steamed or lightly cooked vegetables

Avoid:

Butter- or cream-laden soups and sauces; pies, tarts and quiches; rich potato dishes

Greek

If you ignore the white bread, fries and other potato side dishes, rice, pasta, battered calamari, fried cheese and filo pastry pies, you can pretty much enjoy the rest; that is, until we come to the sweet finale. Greeks have one of the highest per capita consumption of vegetables in the industrialized world, and by far the greatest per capita consumption of olive oil, rich in healthy monounsaturated fatty acids and antioxidants. Nuts and legumes are also part of the traditional Greek diet and there is substantial scientific evidence that these are extremely good for your health. Lemon is used in virtually everything and, apart from being rich in vitamin C and tasting great, it reduces the GL of foods as well.

Start with the ubiquitous Greek salad but avoid the bread. Greek food offers a tremendous variety of mezze, small dishes that are often served together: tzatziki, hummus and *melitzanosalata* (eggplant purée) are excellent appetizers, together with a few olives. Taramasalata (fish roe salad) is delicious but it is usually based on either soaked white bread or mashed potato, not the ideal choice, but then again it is not eaten as a main dish. As a main course try a lentil- or bean-based stew accompanied by vegetables cooked in olive oil. Grilled meat, fish and chicken are good choices, as are the many stews and casseroles. If you wish to order moussaka, first ask the waiter how it is prepared, as it may contain a layer of potato as well as the ubiquitous eggplant topping; the potato-free version is obviously more low glycemic. Greeks have an extremely sweet tooth, but do not normally eat dessert other than fruit, or fruit with yogurt. Sweet cakes like baklava are usually eaten in the early afternoon with coffee and are obviously not good choices.

Best options:
Tzatziki, hummus, split pea purée, eggplant caviar, baked

lima beans in tomato sauce, cannellini bean soup (*fassoláda*), any of the *laderá* (vegetarian dishes cooked in olive oil), Greek ratatouille, baked or grilled seafood, grilled meat, meat casserole

Avoid:

Breaded calamari, dolmades, fried meatballs, moussaka, sausages, pies

Indian

Indian food has some similarities to Greek food (or vice versa) in that it uses fairly similar main ingredients. Indian food, however, tends to include more hot spices and less herbs than Greek food, and clarified butter (ghee) rather than olive oil is the main fat used for cooking.

Traditional Indian cuisine features lots of vegetables, beans and legumes, as well as meat, poultry and seafood, all of which means it should fit well with the principles of a low-glycemic diet. However, there are some pitfalls to contend with. Indian breads are very tasty but high GI, as are deep-fried snacks such as samosas and *pakoras*—so be prepared to resist. There are also many dishes that have rice mixed through them (biryani and pilau) so avoid these, too (although if you are having an ABC reward meal you can have a little basmati rice as a side dish). The amount of ghee used can be excessive so opt for baked or grilled dishes rather than those that are fried or have butter-based sauces.

To start your meal, opt for a raita rather than pappadams; to follow choose tandoori dishes, stews, kebabs or grilled fish. Dishes cooked in yogurt or tomato are also a good option. There's usually also a good choice of vegetarian dishes based on legumes (dal), as well as side dishes with spinach, okra, eggplant and cauliflower. Indian sweets are at least as problematic as the Greek ones. Try a small portion of ice cream if you must but only if you managed to pass on the naan and rice earlier on.

Best options:
Raita, dal or non-creamy bean dishes, chicken tandoori, chicken or fish *saag*, chicken and lentil curry, grilled fish or shellfish

Avoid:
Naan, chapatis, *pakoras*, pappadams (unless they are grilled), *parathas*, samosas, creamy curries (e.g., *kormas* and *pasandas*), biryani and pilau dishes

Italian

Italian cuisine can fit well with the principles of a low-glycemic diet—as long as you look beyond pizza and pasta. Your first challenge is to avoid white bread appetizers (*grissini*, bruschetta, focaccia); opt instead for a light salad, raw vegetable crudités, a selection of antipasti (the equivalent of mezze in Greece and tapas in Spain) or a clear or bean-and-vegetable-based soup such as minestrone. Do not choose a full portion of pasta as a main course; a small portion is fine as long as this is your ABC meal and you forego any bread, potatoes, rice or dessert (other than fruit). If you're in the mood for pizza as your day's reward meal, make sure it has a thin base and is topped with lots of vegetables and chicken or prawns—not cheese. Also be aware of portion sizes: a standard-sized pizza will feed two people when accompanied by a salad or vegetables. Grilled or roasted fish, poultry and veal are good options, but watch out for rich creamy sauces and if necessary ask for the sauce to be served on the side. Polenta is pretty much equivalent to potatoes, pasta and rice, so treat it accordingly as the C part of your ABC reward meal. Fresh fruit should be your dessert of choice.

Best options:
Antipasti (olives, porcini mushrooms, roasted artichokes, etc.); tomato and mozzarella salad, bean salads and any salads with non-creamy dressings; grilled or roasted fish and shellfish; grilled chicken and veal; *arrabiata*, marinara or *pomodoro* sauces; grilled or steamed vegetables

Avoid:
Breads, breaded vegetables or calamari, salami, thick-crust pizza, pizzas with cheese or pepperoni, gnocchi, risotto, anything with cream or cheese-based sauces

Japanese

Is sushi a good choice? Well, it is and it isn't. The protein part of sushi (i.e., raw fish or shellfish), is the healthy part. The sticky rice underneath is high glycemic and should be treated with caution. Remember your ABC plate models. Sushi on its own does not constitute a balanced ABC meal: think of sushi as an appetizer and the C part of your ABC meal, or opt for sashimi instead, which gives you all the health benefits of fish without the rice.

Avoid deep-fried dishes and instead opt for clear soups and broths, which often feature unusual mushrooms such as shiitake and enoki. Stir-fried and steamed vegetables and beans are a good choice (try the great-tasting adzuki and edamame beans), as are tofu dishes. Shabu-shabu is a healthy and sociable way to eat your meat and vegetables, and you have the fun of cooking them yourself. Other healthy Japanese cooking styles include sukiyaki (simmered) and *teppanyaki* (cooked on a hot griddle). Teriyaki dishes, with their sweet, sticky glaze, and tempura (battered and fried) are less healthy. Try to avoid rice and noodles or eat them sparingly as the C part of an ABC meal.

Best options:

Miso soup, *nabemono*, sashimi, grilled fish and shellfish, steamed and stir-fried vegetables, steamed edamame (fresh soy beans), sukiyaki, *teppanyaki*

Avoid:
Tempura; gyoza dumplings; noodles; deep-fried meat and seafood; sushi, sushi rice

Mexican/Southwestern

If you think that Mexican food is limited to tacos and burritos, well, think again. Typical Mexican food offers a variety of bean dishes plus some delicious grilled fish and chicken dishes. Black bean soup is a great choice, since black beans are far more antioxidant-rich than other beans. Refried beans are not the best option, since they are fried in oil after being cooked. Guacamole and the various salsas made from avocado, tomatoes and onions are excellent starters and side dishes. Quesadillas, although tempting, are not a wise choice. Anything with lashings of cheese and sour cream should be avoided. Also, steer clear of tacos and burritos, unless this is the C part of your ABC reward meal and the chef is happy to go easy on the fattening toppings. Grilled meat, chicken, fish or prawns are good choices— just order a large salad alongside. It is perfectly reasonable to order fajitas and ask the waiter to skip the warm tortillas. Chili *sin carne* (i.e., chili made with beans rather than meat) is excellent, although a mixture of meat and beans is fine, too; just say no to the rice.

Best options:
Black bean soup, gazpacho, ceviche, grilled chicken and seafood, chili made with beans

Avoid:
Nachos, tortillas, burritos, tacos, quesadillas, refried beans, sour cream and cheese toppings

Middle Eastern and Turkish

What I have said about Greek food is pretty applicable to Middle Eastern and Turkish cuisine as well. You will find a variety of low-GL mezze, a lot of dishes based on vegetables, olive oil and lentils, beans and chickpeas. Nuts and seeds are also widely used. Tahini (sesame paste) is found in many dishes, including hummus; baba ghanoush (eggplant caviar) is another common Middle Eastern appetizer. Grilled meat, fish and chicken are very common, usually in the form of kebabs. And there are delicious spicy casseroles and *tagines*, which include fruit such as pears and apricots. If you opt for tabbouleh, couscous or bulgur wheat, be aware that this should form the C part of your ABC reward meal.

Best options:
Broad bean and herb salads; cucumber and yogurt salads; hummus; baked eggplant with tomatoes and chickpeas; marinated lamb and chicken dishes; fish and chicken stews and *tagines*; skewered fish, chicken and meat; sautéed and grilled seafoods

Avoid:
Borek (filled pastries), stuffed vine leaves, sautéed potato, grilled or fried cheese, sausages, meatballs, deep-fried seafood

Tapas bars

Tapas bars and Spanish restaurants—pretty much like Greek, Italian and Middle Eastern restaurants—offer an array of healthy dishes. Small portions and great variety are important positive points. Spanish food is greatly influenced by Middle Eastern and North African cuisines; as well as Mediterranean ingredients such as olive oil, you'll find nuts, vegetables and fruits are all used as main ingredients. Grilled fish, meat and chicken are all excellent choices. Paella, although it contains a wonderful array of seafood, is not your best bet because of the amount of rice it contains. However, there is nothing to prevent you from enjoying the seafood and having just a small amount of the rice (if this is your ABC meal of the day), especially if you eat a large portion of vegetables as well. Rice and potato dishes are not the best choices either, including the famous potato-filled tortilla, or Spanish omelette.

Best options:
Olives marinated in lemon or olive oil, mixed peppers and vegetables with tomato sauce, poached octopus, mussels steamed in wine and herbs, grilled sardines and anchovies,

chicken breast in white wine or garlic, grilled pork loin or lamb, grilled tuna and sea bass, skewered and grilled meats
Avoid:
Breads, deep-fried mixed seafood, croquettes, Spanish omelettes, filo-wrapped prawns, fried potatoes with mayonnaise, pancakes filled with goat's cheese

Thai

Traditional Thai food can be very healthy indeed since the cuisine is based around seafood, meat and tofu and enhanced with herbs and spices. However, most Thai restaurants use a lot of thick sweet sauces, particularly creamy coconut sauces. Rice is also an important part of Thai cuisine, and jasmine rice, a very high-glycemic sticky rice, is commonly used, which is far from ideal. Noodles are another popular dish that should be avoided or kept to a minimum. But there are still many good options to choose from while dining at a Thai restaurant: clear yet aromatic soups, wonderfully spicy salads, stir-fried chicken and seafood and unusual vegetable dishes.

Best options:
Tom yum soup (a hot and spicy soup), thin chicken or seafood soups, vegetable and chicken stir-fries with herbs or lemongrass, fresh spring rolls, spicy meat or prawn salads, papaya salad

Avoid:
Coconut soups and curries, fried spring rolls, prawns and vegetables in filo pastry parcels or purses, prawn toasts, sweet chili sauces, dumplings, crispy and fried noodles, jasmine rice

Steak houses and seafood restaurants
In steak houses, you will have no difficulty making wise choices, as long as you opt for lean cuts of meat such as fillet or rump steak, and trim off any visible fat. Ask the waiter to substitute the side order of potatoes or fries for extra salad or vegetables. Avoid anything deep fried and ask for any sauces and dressings to be served separately.

In seafood restaurants you can indulge easily and wisely, just forego or reduce the quantity of starchy side dishes like potatoes, rice, pasta and bread and increase your serving of vegetables and salads.

Best options:
Lean, grilled fillet steak, sirloin or rump; steamed, grilled or boiled vegetables, green salads (no Caesar-style dressings), grilled fish and shellfish

Avoid:
Bread, rich sauces such as bleu cheese, potato dishes, fries, fishcakes, deep-fried and battered fish and shellfish

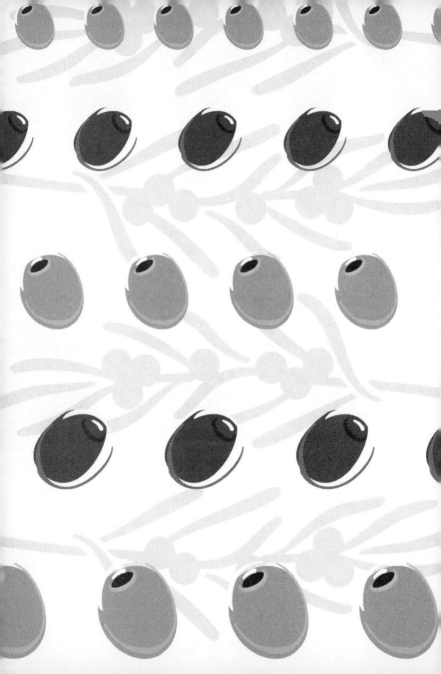

GL Lists:

Alphabetically, by Ascending GL, by Food Group

In this section you'll find the latest GL information for a wide range of foods. The charts are organized in three different configurations to make it easier for you to look up foods in various ways: alphabetically, which makes it easy to find one particular item; by ascending GL, which allows you to identify the foods that fall into the low, medium and high categories; and by food group, which allows you to look at which foods within a group will be most useful for balancing your blood sugar.

It is best to think of carbohydrates as high, medium or low glycemic and not become overly concerned with specific numbers. I consider a GL of 20 or more as high, 11 to 20 as medium, and 10 and below as low.

The first column gives the Glycemic Index (GI). The second column tells you the amount of food containing 50g of carbohydrate: this is the amount of food used in laboratory tests to determine the GI. The third column is what I use to calculate the Glycemic Load (GL) of 100g of food, which you will find in the fourth column.

GL (GLYCEMIC LOAD) LIST ALPHABETICALLY

Foods	GI	Amount of food in grams containing 50g carbohydrate	Carbohydrate per 100g of food	GL per 100g of food
All-Bran (Kellogg's)	42	100	50	21
Apple juice, unsweetened	40	431	12	5
Apples	38	400	13	5
Apples, dried	29	88	57	16
Apricots	57	667	8	4
Apricots, canned, in light syrup	64	316	16	10
Apricots, dried	31	107	47	14
Bagel	72	100	50	36
Baguette	95	100	50	48
Banana	52	250	20	10
Banana bread, made without sugar	55	138	36	20
Barley, pearl	25	179	28	7
Barley porridge/whole-grain barley flour	68	179	28	19
Beans, baked	48	500	10	5
Beans, black, dried, boiled	20	300	17	3
Beans, black-eyed, dried, boiled	42	250	20	8

Beans, cranberry/borlotti, dried, boiled	24	100	12
Beans, fava/broad, boiled	79	364	11
Beans, green, boiled	29	1667	2
Beans, haricot/navy, dried, boiled	38	242	8
Beans, kidney, canned	52	441	6
Beans, kidney, dried, boiled	28	300	5
Beans, lima/canned	36	335	5
Beans, lima/dried, boiled	32	250	6
Beans, mung, dried, boiled	31	441	4
Beans, mung, pressure-cooked	42	441	5
Beans, mung, sprouts	25	441	3
Beans, pinto, dried, boiled	39	288	7
Beans, soy, canned	14	1250	1
Beans, soy, dried, boiled	18	1250	1
Beets	64	571	6
Bran flakes cereal	74	83	44
Bread, flat Middle Eastern	97	94	52
Bread, gluten-free, white	76	100	38
Bread, gluten-free, white, added bran	73	115	32
Bread, hamburger bun	61	100	31
Bread, multigrain	43	108	20

Food of reference: Glucose, GI 100

GL (GLYCEMIC LOAD) LIST ALPHABETICALLY

Foods	GI	Amount of food in grams containing 50g carbohydrate	Carbohydrate per 100g of food	GL per 100g of food
Bread, naan	30	625	8	2
Bread, oatbran	47	83	60	28
Bread, pita	57	88	57	32
Bread, pumpernickel	50	125	40	20
Bread, rice	66	116	43	28
Bread, rye, dark (100% whole-grain)	58	107	47	27
Bread, sourdough, dark, barley	53	75	67	35
Bread, sourdough, white flour	54	107	47	25
Bread, soy and flaxseed	36	166	30	11
Bread, spelt, dark	63	79	63	40
Bread, stone-ground whole-wheat	49	94	53	26
Bread, sunflower and barley	57	151	37	21
Bread, white	70	98	51	36
Bread, white flour, 80% whole-grain	52	75	67	35
Breadfruit	68	222	23	15
Buckwheat	54	250	20	11

Food	GI			
Bulgur wheat	48	288	17	8
Carrot, boiled	58	667	8	4
Carrot, raw	16	500	10	2
Carrot juice	43	543	9	4
Cashews	22	192	26	6
Cassava	46	185	27	12
Cheerios cereal (General Mills)	74	75	67	49
Cherries	22	500	10	2
Chickpeas, canned	42	341	15	6
Chickpeas, chana dal	11	208	24	3
Chickpeas, dried, boiled	28	250	20	6
Chocolate, dark, 70% cocoa solids	22	156	32	7
Chocolate, M&Ms, peanut	33	88	57	19
Chocolate, Mars Bar	65	75	67	43
Chocolate, milk	43	89	56	24
Chocolate, milk (low-sugar, with maltitol)	35	114	44	15
Chocolate, Snickers	55	88	57	31
Chocolate, Twix	44	77	65	29
Coca-Cola	58	481	10	6
Cocoa Krispies (Kellogg's)	77	58	87	67
Corn, fresh	53	234	21	11

Food of reference: Glucose, GI 100

GL (GLYCEMIC LOAD) LIST ALPHABETICALLY

Foods	GI	Amount of food in grams containing 50g carbohydrate	Carbohydrate per 100g of food	GL per 100g of food
Corn chips	63	96	52	33
Cornflakes cereal	81	58	87	70
Couscous, boiled	58	431	12	7
Cranberry juice	56	431	12	6
Crispbread	64	78	64	41
Croissant	67	110	46	31
Dates, dried	103	75	67	69
Doughnut	76	102	49	37
Fanta, orange	68	368	14	9
Figs, dried	61	78	64	39
Frosted Flakes (Kellogg's)	55	58	87	48
Fructose	19	50	100	19
Fruit cocktail, canned	55	375	13	7
Golden raisins	56	66	75	42
Graham crackers	55	73	68	37
Grapefruit	25	545	9	2

Food				
Grapefruit juice, unsweetened	48	625	8	4
Grape-Nuts cereal (Post)	71	71	70	50
Grapes	46	333	15	7
Glucose	100	50	100	100
Honey	55	69	72	40
Hummus	6	300	17	1
Ice cream, low-fat (1.2%–7.1% fat)	43	227	22	9
Ice cream, premium (15% fat)	37	278	18	7
Just Right cereal (Kellogg's)	60	64	78	47
Kiwi fruit	53	500	10	5
Lactose	46	50	100	46
Lentils, green, canned	52	454	11	6
Lentils, green, dried, boiled	30	441	11	3
Lentils, red, dried, boiled	26	417	12	3
Maltose	105	50	100	105
Mango	51	353	14	7
Maple syrup, pure Canadian	54	75	67	36
Marmalade, orange	48	75	67	32
Melon, orange-fleshed	65	1000	5	5
Milk, buttermilk	11	1136	4	0
Milk, low-fat	29	1000	5	1

Food of reference: Glucose, GI 100

GL (GLYCEMIC LOAD) LIST ALPHABETICALLY

Foods	GI	Amount of food in grams containing 50g carbohydrate	Carbohydrate per 100g of food	GL per 100g of food
Milk, nonfat	32	962	5	2
Milk, soy	42	714	7	3
Milk, whole	27	1042	5	1
Millet, boiled	71	208	24	17
Muffin	57	102	49	28
Muesli, unsweetened	49	76	66	32
Mueslix (Kellogg's)	55	79	63	35
Noodles, Chinese vermicelli	58	231	22	13
Noodles, instant	47	225	22	10
Noodles, mung bean/transparent	33	200	25	8
Noodles, rice	61	231	22	13
Nutella chocolate and nut spread	33	83	60	20
Oatcakes	57	79	63	36
Oatmeal, instant	66	481	10	7
Oatmeal, made from oatbran	55	500	10	5
Oatmeal, made from rolled oats	58	568	9	5

Food	GI			
Orange juice, unsweetened	46	481	10	5
Oranges	42	545	9	4
Pancakes, from mix	67	69	73	49
Papaya	59	353	14	8
Parsnip, boiled	97	333	15	15
Pasta, brown rice, boiled	92	237	21	19
Pasta, corn, boiled	54	214	23	13
Pasta, fettuccine (durum wheat), boiled	40	196	26	10
Pasta, gluten-free (maize starch)	54	67	75	40
Pasta, gnocchi (potato-based)	68	188	27	18
Pasta, linguine (durum wheat), boiled	50	196	26	13
Pasta, macaroni, boiled	47	188	27	13
Pasta, spaghetti, al dente	39	191	26	10
Pasta, spaghetti, boiled 10–15 mins	43	188	27	11
Pasta, spaghetti, protein-rich/low-carb, boiled	27	173	29	8
Pasta, spaghetti, whole-wheat, boiled	37	214	23	9
Pastry	59	109	46	27
Peaches	42	545	9	4
Peaches, canned, in juice	38	545	9	3
Peaches, canned, in syrup	57	353	14	8
Peanuts	14	417	12	2

Food of reference: Glucose, GI 100

GL (GLYCEMIC LOAD) LIST ALPHABETICALLY

Foods	GI	Amount of food in grams containing 50g carbohydrate	Carbohydrate per 100g of food	GL per 100g of food
Pears	38	545	9	3
Pears, canned, in juice	43	545	9	4
Peas, green, dried, boiled	22	833	6	1
Peas, green, fresh	48	571	9	4
Pineapple	59	462	11	6
Pineapple juice, unsweetened	46	357	14	6
Pizza (approx. 5 toppings, GI varies from 30—80)	60	185	27	16
Plums	39	500	10	4
Polenta, boiled	68	577	9	6
Popcorn	72	91	55	40
Potato, baked	85	250	20	17
Potato, boiled, peeled	88	417	12	11
Potato, boiled, unpeeled	80	441	11	10
Potato, deep-fried/French fries	75	259	19	15
Potato, instant, mashed	85	375	13	11
Potato, mashed	74	375	13	10

Food			
Potato, new, boiled in skin	57	14	8
Potato, new, canned	63	12	8
Potato, steamed	65	18	18
Potato chips	54	42	23
Powerade	95	16	15
Pretzels	83	67	55
Prunes, pitted, ready-to-eat	29	55	16
Puffed wheat cereal	74	70	52
Pumpernickel bread	50	40	20
Pumpkin, boiled	75	5	4
Quinoa	51	23	12
Raisins	64	73	47
Ravioli, with meat	39	21	8
Rice, basmati, precooked in pouch	57	27	15
Rice, basmati, white	58	25	15
Rice, brown	55	22	12
Rice, jasmine	109	28	31
Rice, parboiled/converted (Uncle Ben's)	47	24	11
Rice, risotto/arborio	69	35	24
Rice, white, long-grain	56	27	15
Rice, white, long-grain, Bangladeshi	38	26	10

Food of reference: Glucose, GI 100

GL (GLYCEMIC LOAD) LIST ALPHABETICALLY

Foods	GI	Amount of food in grams containing 50g carbohydrate	Carbohydrate per 100g of food	GL per 100g of food
Rice, wild	57	238	21	12
Rice cakes	91	60	83	76
Rutabagas	72	750	7	5
Rye, whole-grain, boiled	34	66	76	26
Scones	92	139	36	33
Shredded Wheat cereal	75	76	66	49
Special K (Kellogg's)	54	71	70	38
Sponge cake	54	95	53	29
Sports drink, Gatorade	78	833	6	5
Strawberry jam	51	73	69	35
Strawberries	40	2000	3	1
Sugar (sucrose)	68	50	100	68
Sweet potatoes, cooked	61	268	19	11
Taco shells, corn	68	83	60	41
Tomato juice	38	1389	4	1
Tortilla, flour	52	104	48	25

Food				
Watermelon	72	1000	5	4
Wheaties cereal (General Mills)	70	79	63	44
Wheat, whole-grain, boiled	41	74	68	28
Yam	66	208	24	16
Yogurt, fat-free, natural, unsweetened	33	625	8	3
Yogurt, fat-free, soy, with fruit and sugar	50	385	13	7
Yogurt, fat-free, with aspartame	14	769	7	1
Yogurt, fat-free, with fruit and sugar	33	323	16	5
Yogurt, low-fat, with fruit and aspartame	14	862	6	1
Yogurt, low-fat, with fruit and sugar	33	303	16	5

Food of reference: Glucose, GI 100

GL (GLYCEMIC LOAD) LIST BY ASCENDING GL

Foods	GI	Amount of food in grams containing 50g carbohydrate	Carbohydrate per 100g of food	GL per 100g of food
Milk, buttermilk	11	1136	4	0
Beans, soy, canned	14	1250	4	1
Beans, soy, dried, boiled	18	1250	4	1
Hummus	6	300	17	1
Milk, low-fat	29	1000	5	1
Milk, whole	27	1042	5	1
Peas, green, dried, boiled	22	833	6	1
Strawberries	40	2000	3	1
Tomato juice	38	1389	4	1
Yogurt, fat-free, with aspartame	14	769	7	1
Yogurt, low-fat, with fruit and aspartame	14	862	6	1
Beans, green, boiled	29	1667	8	2
Bread, naan	30	625	8	2
Carrot, raw	16	500	10	2
Cherries	22	500	10	2
Grapefruit	25	545	9	2

Food			
Milk, nonfat	32	962	5	2
Peanuts	14	417	12	2
Beans, black, dried, boiled	20	300	17	3
Beans, mung, sprouts	25	441	11	3
Chickpeas, *chana dal*	11	208	24	3
Lentils, green, dried, boiled	30	441	11	3
Lentils, red, dried, boiled	26	417	12	3
Milk, soy	42	714	7	3
Peaches, canned, in juice	38	545	9	3
Pears	38	545	9	3
Yogurt, fat-free, natural, unsweetened	33	625	8	3
Apricots	57	667	8	4
Beans, mung, dried, boiled	31	441	11	4
Carrot, boiled	58	667	8	4
Carrot juice	43	543	9	4
Grapefruit juice, unsweetened	48	625	8	4
Oranges	42	545	9	4
Peaches	42	545	9	4
Pears, canned, in juice	43	545	9	4
Peas, green, fresh	48	571	9	4
Plums	39	500	10	4

Food of reference: Glucose, GI 100

GL (GLYCEMIC LOAD) LIST BY ASCENDING GL

Foods	GI	Amount of food in grams containing 50g carbohydrate	Carbohydrate per 100g of food	GL per 100g of food
Pumpkin, boiled	75	1000	5	4
Watermelon	72	1000	5	4
Apple juice, unsweetened	40	431	12	5
Apples	38	400	13	5
Beans, baked	48	500	10	5
Beans, kidney, dried, boiled	28	300	17	5
Beans, lima, canned	36	335	15	5
Beans, mung, pressure-cooked	42	441	11	5
Kiwi fruit	53	500	10	5
Melon, orange-fleshed	65	1000	5	5
Oatmeal, made from oatbran	55	500	10	5
Oatmeal, made from rolled oats	58	568	9	5
Orange juice, unsweetened	46	481	10	5
Sports drink, Gatorade	78	833	6	5
Rutabagas	72	750	7	5
Yogurt, fat-free, with fruit and sugar	33	323	16	5

Food		
Yogurt, low-fat, with fruit and sugar	33	303	5
Beans, kidney, canned	52	441	6
Beans, lima, dried, boiled	32	250	6
Beets	64	571	6
Cashews	22	192	6
Chickpeas, canned	42	341	6
Chickpeas, dried, boiled	28	250	6
Coca-Cola	58	481	6
Cranberry juice	56	431	6
Lentils, green, canned	52	454	6
Pineapple	59	462	6
Pineapple juice, unsweetened	46	357	6
Polenta, boiled	68	577	6
Barley, pearl	25	179	7
Beans, pinto, dried, boiled	39	288	7
Chocolate, dark, 70% cocoa solids	22	156	7
Couscous, boiled	58	431	7
Fruit cocktail, canned	55	375	7
Grapes	46	333	7
Ice cream, premium (15% fat)	37	278	7
Oatmeal, instant	66	481	7

Food of reference: Glucose, GI 100

GL (GLYCEMIC LOAD) LIST BY ASCENDING GL

Foods	GI	Amount of food in grams containing 50g carbohydrate	Carbohydrate per 100g of food	GL per 100g of food
Mango	51	353	14	7
Yogurt, fat-free, soy, with fruit and sugar	50	385	13	7
Beans, black-eyed, dried, boiled	42	250	20	8
Beans, haricot/navy, dried, boiled	38	242	21	8
Bulgur wheat	48	288	17	8
Noodles, mung bean/transparent	33	200	25	8
Papaya	59	353	14	8
Pasta, spaghetti, protein-rich/low-carb, boiled	27	173	29	8
Peaches, canned, in syrup	57	353	14	8
Potato, new, boiled in skin	57	357	14	8
Potato, new, canned	63	417	12	8
Ravioli, with meat	39	237	21	8
Fanta, orange	68	368	14	9
Ice cream, low-fat (1.2%–7.1% fat)	43	227	22	9
Pasta, spaghetti, whole-wheat, boiled	37	214	23	9
Apricots, canned, in light syrup	64	316	16	10

Food				
Banana	52	250	20	10
Noodles, instant	47	225	22	10
Pasta, fettuccine (durum wheat), boiled	40	196	26	10
Pasta, spaghetti, al dente	39	191	26	10
Potato, boiled, unpeeled	80	441	11	10
Potato, mashed	74	375	13	10
Rice, white, long-grain, Bangladeshi	38	192	26	10
Beans, fava/broad, boiled	79	364	14	11
Bread, soy and flaxseed	36	166	30	11
Buckwheat	54	250	20	11
Corn, fresh	53	234	21	11
Pasta, spaghetti, boiled 10–15 mins	43	188	27	11
Potato, boiled, peeled	88	417	12	11
Potato, instant, mashed	85	375	13	11
Rice, parboiled/converted (Uncle Ben's)	47	208	24	11
Sweet potatoes, cooked	61	268	19	11
Beans, cranberry/borlotti, dried, boiled	24	100	50	12
Cassava	46	185	27	12
Quinoa	51	217	23	12
Rice, brown	55	227	22	12
Rice, wild	57	238	21	12

Food of reference: Glucose, GI 100

GL (GLYCEMIC LOAD) LIST BY ASCENDING GL

Foods	GI	Amount of food in grams containing 50g carbohydrate	Carbohydrate per 100g of food	GL per 100g of food
Noodles, Chinese vermicelli	58	231	22	13
Noodles, rice	61	231	22	13
Pasta, corn, boiled	54	214	23	13
Pasta, linguine (durum wheat), boiled	50	196	26	13
Pasta, macaroni, boiled	47	188	27	13
Apricots, dried	31	107	47	14
Breadfruit	68	222	23	15
Chocolate, milk (low-sugar, with maltitol)	35	114	44	15
Parsnip, boiled	97	333	15	15
Potato, deep-fried/French fries	75	259	19	15
Powerade	95	312	16	15
Rice, basmati, precooked in pouch	57	185	27	15
Rice, basmati, white	58	197	25	15
Rice, white, long-grain	56	183	27	15
Apples, dried	29	88	57	16
Pizza (approx. 5 toppings, GI varies from 30–80)	60	185	27	16

Prunes, pitted, ready-to-eat	29	55	91	16
Yam	66	24	208	16
Millet, boiled	71	24	208	17
Potato, baked	85	20	250	17
Pasta, gnocchi (potato-based)	68	27	188	18
Potato, steamed	65	18	278	18
Barley porridge/whole-grain barley flour	68	28	179	19
Chocolate, M&Ms, peanut	33	57	88	19
Fructose	19	100	50	19
Pasta, brown rice, boiled	92	21	237	19
Banana bread, made without sugar	55	36	138	20
Bread, multigrain	43	46	108	20
Bread, pumpernickel	50	40	125	20
Nutella chocolate and nut spread	33	60	83	20
All-Bran (Kellogg's)	42	50	100	21
Bread, sunflower and barley	57	37	151	21
Potato chips	54	42	102	23
Chocolate, milk	43	56	89	24
Rice, risotto/arborio	69	35	143	24
Bread, sourdough, white flour	54	47	107	25
Tortilla, Mexican	52	48	104	25

Food of reference: Glucose, GI 100

GL (GLYCEMIC LOAD) LIST BY ASCENDING GL

Foods	GI	Amount of food in grams containing 50g carbohydrate	Carbohydrate per 100g of food	GL per 100g of food
Bread, stone-ground whole-wheat	49	94	53	26
Rye, whole-grain, boiled	34	66	76	26
Bread, rye, dark (100% whole-grain)	58	107	47	27
Pastry	59	109	46	27
Bread, oatbran	47	83	60	28
Bread, rice	66	116	43	28
Muffin	57	102	49	28
Wheat, whole-grain, boiled	41	74	68	28
Chocolate, Twix	44	77	65	29
Sponge cake	54	95	53	29
Bread, hamburger bun	61	100	50	31
Chocolate, Snickers	55	88	57	31
Croissant	67	110	46	31
Rice, jasmine	109	179	28	31
Bread, gluten-free, white, added bran	73	115	43	32
Bread, pita	57	88	57	32

Food				
Marmalade, orange	48	75	67	32
Muesli, unsweetened	49	76	66	32
Corn chips	63	96	52	33
Scones	92	139	36	33
Bread, sourdough, dark, barley	53	75	67	35
Bread, white flour, 80% whole-grain	52	75	67	35
Mueslix (Kellogg's)	55	79	63	35
Strawberry jam	51	73	69	35
Bagel	72	100	50	36
Bread, white	70	98	51	36
Maple syrup, pure Canadian	54	75	67	36
Oatcakes	57	79	63	36
Doughnut	76	102	49	37
Graham crackers	55	73	68	37
Bread, gluten-free, white	76	100	50	38
Special K (Kellogg's)	54	71	70	38
Figs, dried	61	78	64	39
Bread, spelt, dark	63	79	63	40
Honey	55	69	72	40
Pasta, gluten-free (maize starch)	54	67	75	40
Popcorn	72	91	55	40

Food of reference: Glucose, GI 100

GL (GLYCEMIC LOAD) LIST BY ASCENDING GL

Foods	GI	Amount of food in grams containing 50g carbohydrate	Carbohydrate per 100g of food	GL per 100g of food
Crispbread	64	78	64	41
Taco shells, corn	68	83	60	41
Golden raisins	56	66	75	42
Chocolate, Mars Bar	65	75	67	43
Bran flakes cereal	74	83	60	44
Wheaties cereal (General Mills)	70	79	63	44
Lactose	46	50	100	46
Just Right cereal (Kellogg's)	60	64	78	47
Raisins	64	68	73	47
Baguette	95	100	50	48
Frosted Flakes (Kellogg's)	55	58	87	48
Cheerios cereal (General Mills)	74	75	67	49
Pancakes, from mix	67	69	73	49
Shredded Wheat cereal	75	76	66	49
Grape-Nuts cereal (Post)	71	71	70	50
Bread, flat Middle Eastern	97	94	53	52

Food			
Puffed wheat cereal	74	71	70	52
Pretzels	83	75	67	55
Cocoa Krispies (Kellogg's)	77	58	87	67
Sugar (sucrose)	68	50	100	68
Dates, dried	103	75	67	69
Cornflakes cereal	81	58	87	70
Rice cakes	91	60	83	76
Glucose	100	50	100	100
Maltose	105	50	100	105

GL (GLYCEMIC LOAD) LIST BY FOOD GROUP

Foods	GI	Amount of food in grams containing 50g carbohydrate	Carbohydrate per 100g of food	GL per 100g of food
BAKED GOODS				
Banana bread, made without sugar	55	138	36	20
Croissant	67	110	46	31
Doughnut	76	102	49	37
Graham crackers	55	73	68	37
Muffin	57	102	49	28
Pancakes, from mix	67	69	73	49
Pastry	59	109	46	27
Pizza (approx. 5 toppings, GI varies from 30 to 80)	60	185	27	16
Scones	92	139	36	33
Sponge cake	54	95	53	29
Taco shells, corn	68	83	60	41
Tortilla, Mexican	52	104	48	25

BEANS AND LEGUMES

Beans, baked	48	500	10	5
Beans, black, dried, boiled	20	300	17	3
Beans, black-eyed, dried, boiled	42	250	20	8
Beans, cranberry/borlotti, dried, boiled	24	100	50	12
Beans, fava/broad, boiled	79	364	14	11
Beans, green, boiled	29	1667	8	2
Beans, haricot/navy, dried, boiled	38	242	21	8
Beans, kidney, canned	52	441	11	6
Beans, kidney, dried, boiled	28	300	17	5
Beans, lima, canned	36	335	15	5
Beans, lima, dried, boiled	32	250	20	6
Beans, mung, dried, boiled	31	441	11	4
Beans, mung, pressure-cooked	42	441	11	5
Beans, mung, sprouts	25	441	11	3
Beans, pinto, dried, boiled	39	288	17	7
Beans, soy, canned	14	1250	4	1
Beans, soy, dried, boiled	18	1250	4	1
Chickpeas, *chana* dal	11	208	24	3
Chickpeas, canned	42	341	15	6
Chickpeas, dried, boiled	28	250	20	6

Food of reference: Glucose, GI 100

GL (GLYCEMIC LOAD) LIST BY FOOD GROUP

Foods	GI	Amount of food in grams containing 50g carbohydrate	Carbohydrate per 100g of food	GL per 100g of food
Hummus	6	300	17	1
Lentils, green, canned	52	454	11	6
Lentils, green, dried, boiled	30	441	11	3
Lentils, red, dried, boiled	26	417	12	3
BREADS				
Bagel	72	100	50	36
Baguette	95	100	50	48
Bread, flat Middle Eastern	97	94	53	52
Bread, gluten-free, white	76	100	50	38
Bread, gluten-free, white, added bran	73	115	43	32
Bread, hamburger bun	61	100	50	31
Bread, multigrain	43	108	46	20
Bread, naan	30	625	8	2
Bread, oatbran	47	83	60	28
Bread, pita	57	88	57	32

Bread, pumpernickel	50	125	40	20
Bread, rice	66	116	43	28
Bread, rye, dark (100% whole-grain)	58	107	47	27
Bread, sourdough, dark, barley	53	75	67	35
Bread, sourdough, white flour	54	107	47	25
Bread, soy and flaxseed	36	166	30	11
Bread, spelt, dark	63	79	63	40
Bread, stone-ground whole-wheat	49	94	53	26
Bread, sunflower and barley	57	151	37	21
Bread, white	70	98	51	36
Bread, white flour, 80% whole-grain	52	75	67	35

BREAKFAST CEREALS

All-Bran (Kellogg's)	42	100	50	21
Bran flakes cereal	74	83	60	44
Cheerios cereal (General Mills)	74	75	67	49
Cocoa Krispies (Kellogg's)	77	58	87	67
Cornflakes cereal	81	58	87	70
Frosted Flakes (Kellogg's)	55	58	87	48
Grape-Nuts cereal (Post)	71	71	70	50
Just Right cereal (Kellogg's)	60	64	78	47

Food of reference: Glucose, GI 100

GL (GLYCEMIC LOAD) LIST BY FOOD GROUP

Foods	GI	Amount of food in grams containing 50g carbohydrate	Carbohydrate per 100g of food	GL per 100g of food
Mueslix (Kellogg's)	55	79	63	35
Muesli, unsweetened	49	76	66	32
Oatmeal, instant	66	481	10	7
Oatmeal, made from oatbran	55	500	10	5
Oatmeal, made from rolled oats	58	568	9	5
Puffed wheat cereal	74	71	70	52
Shredded Wheat cereal	75	76	66	49
Special K (Kellogg's)	54	71	70	38
Wheaties cereal (General Mills)	70	79	63	44

CHOCOLATE

Foods	GI	Amount of food in grams containing 50g carbohydrate	Carbohydrate per 100g of food	GL per 100g of food
Chocolate, dark, 70% cocoa solids	22	156	32	7
Chocolate, M&Ms, peanut	33	88	57	19
Chocolate, Mars	65	75	67	43
Chocolate, milk	43	89	56	24
Chocolate, milk (low-sugar, with maltitol)	35	114	44	15

Food	GI			
Chocolate, Snickers	55	88	57	31
Chocolate, Twix	44	77	65	29

DAIRY PRODUCTS

Food				
Ice cream, low-fat (1.2%–7.1% fat)	43	227	22	9
Ice cream, premium (15% fat)	37	278	18	7
Milk, buttermilk	11	1136	4	0
Milk, low-fat	29	1000	5	1
Milk, nonfat	32	962	5	2
Milk, whole	27	1042	5	1
Yogurt, fat-free, natural, unsweetened	33	625	8	3
Yogurt, fat-free, soy, with fruit and sugar	50	385	13	7
Yogurt, fat-free, with aspartame	14	769	7	1
Yogurt, fat-free, with fruit and sugar	33	323	16	5
Yogurt, low-fat, with fruit and aspartame	14	862	6	1
Yogurt, low-fat, with fruit and sugar	33	303	16	5

DRINKS

Food				
Apple juice, unsweetened	40	431	12	5
Carrot juice	43	543	9	4
Coca-Cola	58	481	10	6

Food of reference: Glucose, GI 100

GL (GLYCEMIC LOAD) LIST BY FOOD GROUP

Foods	GI	Amount of food in grams containing 50g carbohydrate	Carbohydrate per 100g of food	GL per 100g of food
Cranberry juice	56	431	12	6
Fanta, orange	68	368	14	9
Grapefruit juice, unsweetened	48	625	8	4
Milk, soy	42	714	7	3
Orange juice, unsweetened	46	481	10	5
Pineapple juice, unsweetened	46	357	14	6
Powerade	95	312	16	15
Tomato juice	38	1389	4	1
Sports drink, Gatorade	78	833	6	5
FRUIT				
Apples	38	400	13	5
Apples, dried	29	88	57	16
Apricots	57	667	8	4

Food				
Apricots, canned, in light syrup	64	316	16	10
Apricots, dried	31	107	47	14
Banana	52	250	20	10
Breadfruit	68	222	23	15
Cherries	22	500	10	2
Dates, dried	103	75	67	69
Figs, dried	61	78	64	39
Fruit cocktail, canned	55	375	13	7
Golden raisins	56	66	75	42
Grapefruit	25	545	9	2
Grapes	46	333	15	7
Kiwi fruit	53	500	10	5
Mango	51	353	14	7
Melon, orange-fleshed	65	1000	5	5
Oranges	42	545	9	4
Papaya	59	353	14	8
Peaches	42	545	9	4
Peaches, canned, in juice	38	545	9	3
Peaches, canned, in syrup	57	353	14	8
Pears	38	545	9	3
Pears, canned, in juice	43	545	9	4

Food of reference: Glucose, GI 100

GL (GLYCEMIC LOAD) LIST BY FOOD GROUP

Foods	GI	Amount of food in grams containing 50g carbohydrate	Carbohydrate per 100g of food	GL per 100g of food
Pineapple	59	462	11	6
Plums	39	500	10	4
Prunes, pitted, ready-to-eat	29	91	55	16
Raisins	64	68	73	47
Strawberries	40	2000	3	1
Watermelon	72	1000	5	4
GRAINS				
Barley, pearl	25	179	28	7
Barley porridge/whole-grain barley flour	68	179	28	19
Buckwheat	54	250	20	11
Bulgur wheat	48	288	17	8
Couscous, boiled	58	431	12	7
Millet, boiled	71	208	24	17
Polenta, boiled	68	577	9	6
Quinoa	51	217	23	12

Rice, basmati, precooked in pouch	57	185	27	15
Rice, basmati, white	58	197	25	15
Rice, brown	55	227	22	12
Rice, jasmine	109	179	28	31
Rice, parboiled/converted (Uncle Ben's)	47	208	24	11
Rice, risotto/arborio	69	143	35	24
Rice, white, long-grain	56	183	27	15
Rice, white, long-grain, Bangladeshi	38	192	26	10
Rice, wild	57	238	21	12
Rye, whole-grain, boiled	34	66	76	26
Wheat, whole-grain, boiled	41	74	68	28

NOODLES AND PASTA

Noodles, Chinese vermicelli	58	231	22	13
Noodles, instant	47	225	22	10
Noodles, mung bean/transparent	33	200	25	8
Noodles, rice	61	231	22	13
Pasta, brown rice, boiled	92	237	21	19
Pasta, corn, boiled	54	214	23	13
Pasta, fettuccine (durum wheat), boiled	40	196	26	10
Pasta, gluten-free (maize starch)	54	67	75	40

Food of reference: Glucose, GI 100

GL (GLYCEMIC LOAD) LIST BY FOOD GROUP

Foods	GI	Amount of food in grams containing 50g carbohydrate	Carbohydrate per 100g of food	GL per 100g of food
Pasta, gnocchi (potato-based)	68	188	27	18
Pasta, linguine (durum wheat), boiled	50	196	26	13
Pasta, macaroni, boiled	47	188	27	13
Pasta, spaghetti, al dente	39	191	26	10
Pasta, spaghetti, boiled 10–15 mins	43	188	27	11
Pasta, spaghetti, protein-rich/low-carb, boiled	27	173	29	8
Pasta, spaghetti, whole-wheat, boiled	37	214	23	9
Ravioli, with meat	39	237	21	8
NUTS				
Cashews	22	192	26	6
Peanuts	14	417	12	2
SAVORY SNACKS				
Corn chips	63	96	52	33
Crispbread	64	78	64	41

Food				
Oatcakes	57	79	63	36
Popcorn	72	91	55	40
Pretzels	83	75	67	55
Rice cakes	91	60	83	76
SPREADS				
Maple syrup, pure Canadian	54	75	67	36
Marmalade, orange	48	75	67	32
Nutella chocolate and nut spread	33	83	60	20
Strawberry jam	51	73	69	35
SUGARS				
Fructose	19	50	100	19
Glucose	100	50	100	100
Honey	55	69	72	40
Lactose	46	50	100	46
Maltose	105	50	100	105
Sugar (sucrose)	68	50	100	68

Food of reference: Glucose, GI 100

GL (GLYCEMIC LOAD) LIST BY FOOD GROUP

Foods	GI	Amount of food in grams containing 50g carbohydrate	Carbohydrate per 100g of food	GL per 100g of food
VEGETABLES				
Beets	64	571	9	6
Carrot, boiled	58	667	8	4
Carrot, raw	16	500	10	2
Cassava	46	185	27	12
Corn, fresh	53	234	21	11
Parsnip, boiled	97	333	15	15
Peas, green, dried, boiled	22	833	6	1
Peas, green, fresh	48	571	9	4
Potato, baked	85	250	20	17
Potato, boiled, unpeeled	80	441	11	10
Potato, deep-fried/French fries	75	259	19	15
Potato, instant, mashed	85	375	13	11
Potato, mashed	74	375	13	10
Potato, new, boiled in skin	57	357	14	8
Potato, new, canned	63	417	12	8

Potato, steamed	65	278	18	18
Potato chips	54	102	42	23
Pumpkin, boiled	75	1000	5	4
Rutabagas	72	750	7	5
Sweet potatoes, cooked	61	268	19	11
Yam	66	208	24	16

Food of reference: Glucose, GI 100

Index